first place 4health

Bible Study Series

a thankful
heart

Christin Ditchfield

Published by Gospel Light
Ventura, California, U.S.A.
www.gospellight.com
Printed in the U.S.A.

Caution: The information contained in this book is intended to be solely for
informational and educational purposes. It is assumed that the First Place 4 Health
participant will consult a medical or health professional before beginning this or
any other weight-loss or physical fitness program.

Library of Congress Cataloging-in-Publication Data
A thankful heart.
p. cm. — (First place 4 health Bible study series)
ISBN 978-0-8307-6434-1 (trade paper)
1. Gratitude—Religious aspects—Christianity—Textbooks.
2. Gratitude—Biblical teaching. I. Gospel Light Publications (Firm)
BV4647.G8T437 2012
248.4071—dc23
2012031536

Rights for publishing this book outside the U.S.A. or in non-English
languages are administered by Gospel Light Worldwide, an international
not-for-profit ministry. For additional information, please visit
www.glww.org, email info@glww.org, or write to Gospel Light Worldwide,
1957 Eastman Avenue, Ventura, CA 93003, U.S.A.

To order copies of this book and other First Place 4 Health products
in bulk quantities, please contact us at 1-800-727-5223. You can also
order copies from Gospel Light at 1-800-446-7735.

contents

about the author

Christin Ditchfield is host of the internationally syndicated radio program *Take It To Heart!*® Using real-life stories, rich word pictures, biblical illustrations, and touches of humor, she calls believers to enthusiastically seek after God, giving them practical tools to help deepen their personal relationships with Christ. Christin is an accomplished educator, popular conference speaker, and author of more than 60 books, including *A Family Guide to the Bible* and the First Place 4 Health studies *A New Beginning* and *Living for Christ*. She holds a master's degree in Biblical Theology from Southwestern University. For more information about Christin and her ministry, visit her website at www.TakeItToHeartRadio.com.

foreword

My introduction to Bible study came when I joined First Place in March 1981. I had been attending church since I was a small child, but the extent of my study of the Bible had been reading my Sunday School quarterly on Saturday night. On Sunday morning, I would listen to my Sunday School teacher as she taught God's Word to me. During the worship service, I would listen to our pastor as he taught God's Word to me. Frankly, the idea of digging out the truths of the Bible for myself had never entered my mind.

Perhaps you are right where I was back in 1981. If so, you are in for a blessing you never dreamed possible. As you start studying the truths of the Bible for yourself through the First Place 4 Health Bible studies, you will see God begin to open your understanding of His Word.

Almost every First Place 4 Health member I have talked with about the program says, "The weight loss is wonderful, but the most important thing I have received from my association with First Place 4 Health is learning to study God's Word." The First Place 4 Health Bible studies are designed to be done on a daily basis. As you work through each day's study (which will take 15 to 20 minutes to complete), you will be discovering the deep truths of God's Word. A part of each week's study will also include a Bible memory verse for the week.

There are many in-depth Bible studies on the market. The First Place 4 Health Bible studies are not designed for the purpose of in-depth study, but are designed to be used in conjunction with the rest of the program to bring balance into your life. Our desire is for each member to begin having a personal quiet time with God each day. This time alone with God should include a time of prayer, Bible reading and Bible study. Having a quiet time is a daily discipline that will bring the rich rewards of balance, which is something we all need.

God bless you as you begin this exciting journey toward a balanced life. God will richly bless your efforts to give Him first place in your life. Remember Matthew 6:33: "But seek first his kingdom and his righteousness, and all these things will be given to you as well."

Carole Lewis, First Place 4 Health National Director

introduction

First Place 4 Health is a Christ-centered health program that emphasizes balance in the physical, mental, emotional and spiritual areas of life. The First Place 4 Health program is meant to be a daily process. As we learn to keep Christ first in our lives, we will find that He is the One who satisfies our hunger and our every need.

This Bible study is designed to be used in conjunction with the First Place 4 Health program but can be beneficial for anyone interested in obtaining a balanced lifestyle. The Bible study has been created in a five-day format, with the last two days reserved for reflection on the material studied. Keep in mind that the ultimate goal of studying the Bible is not only for knowledge but also for application and a changed life. Don't feel anxious if you can't seem to find the *correct* answer. Many times, the Word will speak differently to different people, depending on where they are in their walk with God and the season of life they are experiencing. Be prepared to discuss with your fellow First Place 4 Health members what you learned that week through your study.

There are some additional components included with this study that will be helpful as you pursue the goal of giving Christ first place in every area of your life:

- **Group Prayer Request Form:** This form is at the end of each week's study. You can use this to record any special requests that might be given in class.

- **Leader Discussion Guide:** This discussion guide is provided to help the First Place 4 Health leader guide a group through this Bible study. It includes ideas for facilitating a First Place 4 Health class discussion for each week of the Bible study.

- **Two Weeks of Menu Plans with Recipes:** There are 14 days of meals, and all are interchangeable. Each day totals 1,400 to 1,500 calories and includes snacks. Instructions are given for those who need more calories. An accompanying grocery list includes items needed for each week of meals.

- **First Place 4 Health Member Survey:** Fill this out and bring it to your first meeting. This information will help your leader know your interests and talents.

- **Personal Weight and Measurement Record:** Use this form to keep a record of your weight loss. Record any loss or gain on the chart after the weigh-in at each week's meeting.

- **Weekly Prayer Partner Forms:** Fill out this form before class and place it into a basket during the class meeting. After class, you will draw out a prayer request form, and this will be your prayer partner for the week. Try to call or email the person sometime before the next class meeting to encourage that person.

- **Live It Trackers:** Your Live It Tracker is to be completed at home and turned in to your leader at your weekly First Place 4 Health meeting. The Tracker is designed to help you practice mindfulness and stay accountable with regard to your eating and exercise habits. Step-by-step instructions for how to use the Live It Tracker are provided in the *Member's Guide*.

- **Let's Count Our Miles!** A worthy goal we encourage is for you to complete 100 miles of exercise during your 12 weeks in First Place 4 Health. There are many activities listed on pages 253-254 that count toward your goal of 100 miles. When you complete a mile of activity, mark off the box listed on the Hundred Mile Club chart located on the inside of the back cover.

- **Scripture Memory Cards:** These cards have been designed so you can use them while exercising. It is suggested that you punch a hole in the upper left corner and place the cards on a ring. You may want to take the cards in the car or to work so you can practice each week's Scripture memory verse throughout the day.

- **Scripture Memory CD:** All 10 Scripture memory verses have been put to music at an exercise tempo in the CD at the back of this study. Use this CD when exercising or even when you are just driving in your car. The words of Scripture are often easier to memorize when accompanied by music.

welcome to
A Thankful Heart

At your first group meeting for this session of First Place 4 Health, you will meet your fellow members, get an overview of your materials and find out what you can expect at weekly meetings. The majority of your class time will be spent learning about the four-sided person concept, the Live It Food Plan, and how change begins from the inside out. You will also have a chance to ask any questions about how to get the most out of First Place 4 Health. If possible, complete the Member Survey on page 203 before your first group meeting. The information that you give will help your leader tailor the next 12 weeks to the needs of the whole group.

Each weekly meeting begins with a weigh-in for members. This will allow you to track your progress over the 12-week session. Your Week One weigh-in/measurement will establish a baseline of comparison so that you can set healthy goals for this session. If you are apprehensive about weighing in every week, talk with your group leader about your concerns. He or she will have some options for you to consider that will make the weigh-in activity encouraging rather than stressful.

The day after your first meeting, begin Week Two of this Bible study. This study is a companion to *A Thankful Heart* by Carole Lewis, so it is recommended that you read that book before beginning. This session, you and your group will discover how having a thankful heart will transform every area of your life and bring the victory in Christ you have been longing for. As you open yourself to the truth of Scripture and share your hopes and struggles with the members of your group during the next 12 weeks, you'll find yourself becoming the healthy child of God you are designed to be!

thankful
for each moment

SCRIPTURE MEMORY VERSE

*Those God foreknew he also predestined to be
conformed to the likeness of his Son, that
he might be the firstborn among many brothers.*

ROMANS 8:29

There's a verse in the Bible that contains the key to living an extraordinary, victorious, joy-filled life: "Give thanks in all circumstances, for this is God's will for you in Christ Jesus" (1 Thessalonians 5:18). When you think about it, it's a pretty radical concept. As human beings, we're not naturally thankful. Author Ann Voskamp observes:

> From all of our beginnings, we keep reliving the Garden story. Satan, he wanted more. More power, more glory. Ultimately, in his essence, Satan is an ingrate. And he sinks his venom into the heart of Eden. Satan's sin becomes the first sin of all humanity *the sin of ingratitude.* Adam and Eve are simply, painfully, ungrateful for what God gave. Isn't that the catalyst of all my sins? Our fall was, has always been, and always will be, that we aren't satisfied in God and what He gives. We hunger for something more, something other.[1]

When we don't get what we want, our hearts are full of bitterness, anger, frustration and despair. We complain and complain, making ourselves more miserable and spreading that misery to everyone around us!

What we desperately need is a heart transplant. In Ezekiel 36:26, God says, "I will give you a new heart and put a new spirit in you; I will remove from you your heart of stone and give you a heart of flesh." We need to fill our new hearts with gratitude, with thanksgiving. We must consciously look for the positive—all the good things we've been given—and reject the temptation to dwell on the negative—all the things we don't like or don't have.

It's not always easy. We can't do it on our own. But God is ready and willing to help us. Moment by moment, day by day, we can choose to give thanks—and experience His grace, His peace and His joy. Will you make that choice today? "Yesterday is history. Tomorrow is a mystery. Today is God's gift—that's why it is called the present."

Day 1

CHOOSING JESUS

God, help me to realize that every moment You give me is a precious gift I can give back to You. Amen.

Practice this week's memory verse by filling in the blanks below.

Those God _____ he also _____ to be _____ to the _____ of his _____, that _____ might be the _____ among many _____ (Romans 8:29).

Let's read this verse in context. In the *New Living Translation,* Romans 8:28-30 reads:

And we know that God causes everything to work together for the good of those who love God and are called according to his purpose for them. For God knew his people in advance, and he chose them to become like his Son, so that his Son would be the firstborn among many brothers and sisters. And having chosen them, he called them to come to him. And having called them, he gave them right standing with himself. And having given them right standing, He gave them his glory.

According to Romans 5:8, how did God give us "right standing with himself"? Why did God do this?

_____

_____

_____

_____

The Bible tells us that we've all been born with a sinful nature—a stubborn self-will that wants its own way in everything. We've all sinned. We've all fallen short of God's righteous and holy standards (see Romans 3:23). Out of ignorance or rebellion, we have disregarded and disobeyed His commands. Because God is just, He must hold us accountable—our sins must be paid for. And the penalty is death, physical and spiritual—eternal separation from God (see Romans 6:23).

Because God is merciful, however, He sent His precious Son, Jesus, to lay down His life for us, to pay the penalty for our sins and take the punishment in our place. He died on the cross and then was raised from the dead in power and glory. He lives today, and because He lives, so can we (see Galatians 2:20). According to John 1:12, what special right, or privilege, did Jesus purchase for us with His blood?

_____

_____

_____

_____

How do we receive that right, or privilege?

_____

_____

_____

_____

Take a moment to remember when this precious truth first became a reality for you—when you first became a child of God. Why did you decide to open your heart to Jesus? What has this meant to you? How has it impacted the way you live your life today?

_____

_____

_____

Thank You, Jesus, for loving me so much that You couldn't leave me lost in sin. Let the life I live be a reflection of my love for You. Amen.

Day 2 CHOOSING LIFE

Lord, I'm so thankful for these moments I get to spend with You. Speak to my heart today and every day. Amen.

Reflecting on Romans 8:29, this week's memory verse, First Place 4 Health National Director Carole Lewis says:

> God has an amazing plan for us, and He uses the moments of our lives to fulfill His plan. God wants us to become like His Son, Jesus Christ. He wants to transform us—to change us—into people who live and act as Christ lives. God isn't content to leave us wallowing in our sins—He loves us too much for that. He wants to give us more than we could dare to ask or imagine. He wants to make us like Christ. Developing a thankful heart is part of God's purpose for our moments. God wants us to look more and more like Christ every day we live. God wants us to think like Jesus, talk like Jesus and, yes, to act like Jesus. God wants us all to cultivate thankful hearts. God wants us to begin thanking Him in every situation in which we find ourselves.[2]

Look up John 10:10. How did Jesus describe the life to which He has called us?

_____

_____

_____

The original Greek word used in this verse could also be translated "abundant," "overflowing," "in all its fullness," "far more than before" or "more and better than they ever dreamed of." But it's a choice! We have to choose this life. We have to choose to obey. As Carole Lewis states:

> When it comes to the transforming work God does in our lives, He allows us the wonderful privilege of being a part of this work. God never drags us kicking and screaming to somewhere we don't want to go. He gives us free will—the ability to say yes and no, the capacity to obey or disobey.[3]

What did God tell His people in Deuteronomy 30:19?

_____

_____

_____

According to 1 John 5:3, how do we show what we have chosen?

_____

_____

_____

Read Psalm 112. Although all of God's commands may not always be easy to obey, how should we feel about obeying them? What will be the result (see verse 1)?

_____

_____

_____

_____

What sort of blessings will we receive (see verses 3-6)?

_____

_____

_____

What should our reaction be during times of trouble? Why are we able to react this way (see verses 7-8)?

_____

_____

_____

_____

If we want to be more like Jesus and experience the life He has called us to—in all its fullness—we must make a choice. We must choose to trust and obey Him. We must choose to give thanks. It's an act of faith—one that will change us forever.

> *Jesus, I choose You. I choose life. I choose hope. I choose love. I choose faith. I choose obedience. Amen.*

Day 3 — CHOOSING THANKS

> *Jesus, be with me today. Help me to see Your hand in everything that comes my way. I choose to have a thankful heart. Amen.*

What command are we given in 1 Thessalonians 5:18?

_____

_____

_____

_____

Read Psalm 34:1. What declaration did the psalmist make?

_____

_____

_____

_____

The word "extol" means to bless, to praise highly, to exalt, to magnify or glorify, or to celebrate. Look up Psalm 71:14-18. According to these verses and the verse you read in Psalms 34, when and how much are we to thank and praise God?

_____

_____

_____

_____

_____

As Carole Lewis states, "We can bring an attitude of thankfulness to any experience; and when we do, it's like a breath of fresh air rushing in and blowing away the dust of decay. Some people possess an attitude of gratitude more naturally than others. But all of us are called to step onto this path. . . . As we learn to cultivate a thankful heart, our grumbling and complaining will cease and be replaced by a spirit that blesses God, blesses those around us and even blesses ourselves."[4]

Interestingly, scientific studies have shown that a thankful heart has as much impact on a person's health as physical exercise. People who choose to be thankful are happier, more optimistic and more energetic. They have lower levels of chronic stress and have fewer physical symptoms of illness and pain. They sleep better. They do better at their endeavors, be they at school or at work. They have stronger relationships with their friends and families. They are more creative; they have better problem-solving skills. They are better able to cope with life's challenges—even tragedies—without succumbing to stress, envy, bitterness or depression.[5] Given this, should we really be surprised to find that what God tells us to do—give thanks—is for our own good?

Look up Deuteronomy 30:11. What else do we learn about God's commandments?

_____

_____

_____

_____

_____

Take a few moments to reflect on the condition of your own heart today. Are you thankful most of the time, some of the time, once in a while or hardly ever? How often do you express your thanks to God and others? How would you like your heart to be?

_____

_____

_____

_____

Father, teach me how to have a truly thankful heart, a grateful heart, a heart full of love for You. Amen.

Day 4 — CHOOSING JOY

Lord, help me to be joyful in hope, patient in affliction, and faithful in prayer. Help me always to be thankful, each and every day. Amen.

Author and speaker Pam Farrel talks about a time when one tragedy or crisis after another had made it almost impossible for her to answer the question, "How are you?" without launching into a long explanation of a lot of discouraging and depressing circumstances. As she prayed about it, God spoke to her heart and reminded her that she had a choice. She could choose to focus on all that was wrong or all that was right. She could count her trials or count her blessings. She could choose to be miserable or to be thankful. She could choose misery or joy. From that moment on, when people asked how she was doing, she answered, "Choosin' joy!" Over time, that joy became a spring of life bubbling out of her.[6] Read Psalm 16:11. Why (or for what) did the psalmist praise God?

_____

_____

_____

_____

Look up Galatians 5:22-23. What are the different fruit of the Spirit—the evidence of God working in our hearts and lives—listed in this passage?

_____

_____

_____

_____

Would you like to see more of this fruit in your life—including joy? Choose to give thanks to God—to express your absolute faith and trust and confidence in Him—for everything He is and everything He does. Your joy will know no bounds! Look up Colossians 2:6-8. Putting our faith in Jesus, trusting in Him, is not a one-time thing. According to these verses, what should we do?

_____

_____

_____

_____

_____

Paul compares our relationship with Christ to that of a plant. How are we rooted in Christ? What do we receive through our roots in Him?

_____

_____

_____

_____

_____

Why are the ways of the world "hollow and deceptive"?

_____

_____

_____

_____

What can you do in your life today to become more rooted, more built up, more alive in Christ? How can your First Place 4 Health group help you do this?

_____

_____

_____

_____

Lord, I thank You for Your love, Your peace, Your patience, Your kindness, Your goodness and Your mercy to me. You alone are my joy. Amen.

Day
5

CHOOSING CHANGE

God, thank You for leading me on this journey. Do a new work in my heart and life every day. Amen.

What would you like to see God accomplish in your life over the next 10 weeks? Do you have a particular objective in mind? Any specific hopes and dreams? Prayerfully consider what God's goals for you might be. Ask Him to help you set a particular goal for each of the following areas of your life. (You may have more than one goal, but for your own sake, try to keep these goals as simple and focused as possible. Think about the next 10 weeks only!)

Physical health

_____

_____

_____

Mental health

_____

_____

_____

Emotional health

_____
_____
_____
_____

Spiritual health

_____
_____
_____

Now list one specific step that you can take toward achieving each of your goals.

Physical health

_____
_____
_____

Mental health

_____
_____
_____

Emotional health

_____
_____
_____

Spiritual health

_____
_____
_____

Looking over these goals, you may feel motivated, energized and inspired. You may also feel some anxiety, worry or fear that you won't be able to achieve them. What encouragement do you find in Psalm 28:7? Paraphrase the verse—write it in your own words—making it personal to you and your journey

_____

_____

_____

_____

Lord, I commit all my plans, my goals, my hopes and dreams to You.
Help me to do my part to bring glory and honor to You. Amen.

Day 6 REFLECTION AND APPLICATION

Thank You, Father, that Your love for us never ceases; Your mercies never come to an end. They are new every morning. Great is Your faithfulness. Amen.

Carole Lewis shares from her own experience that creating—and keeping—a thankfulness journal is one of the best ways to cultivate a thankful heart. Your journal can be a list you keep on a legal pad, in a special notebook or scrapbook, or even with a smartphone app![7] However you choose to record the things you're thankful for, Carole suggests you follow these five tips:

1. Keep it simple. Focus on giving thanks, not processing your feelings or writing out your prayers (have a separate prayer journal for that). Write one or two sentences that start with "I am thankful for . . ." You could also add small photos or drawings or mementos of special occasions.

2. Keep it honest. Don't fake it. Only list things for which you are genuinely thankful. God knows your heart.

3. Keep it personal. Focus on you and your relationship with God. Don't indirectly criticize or judge others, the way the Pharisee did in Luke 18:11, thanking God that he wasn't a sinner like those other people!

4. Keep it specific. Don't just thank God in general terms for His love or faithfulness. Write down specifically what made you thankful for these things, what circumstances reminded you of them.

5. Keep it consistent. Add to your thankfulness journal daily. If you were to list five things you are thankful for each morning and five things each evening, by the end of this study, you'd have thanked God for at least 700 things! If adding 10 entries each day seems too much, try for five a day (total) or even three a day. What a great way to develop an attitude of gratitude![8]

During this session, Day 7 of each week's study will include space for a thankfulness journal entry. You can fill in this entry during the week as the things you're thankful for happen or fill in the entry as a way to review the week. You may choose to use these entries specifically for things you're thankful for that relate to your First Place 4 Health journey, or you may choose to include anything and everything you are thankful for in your life today! For right now as practice, list a few reasons you're thankful for choosing the First Place 4 Health program.

_____

_____

_____

_____

_____

Father, teach me to be thankful for each day—each moment—You have given to me. Help me always to bring glory and honor to You. Amen.

REFLECTION AND APPLICATION

Holy Spirit, please bring to my remembrance all the things that You have taught me this week, all the ways You have shown Your love for me, all the things for which I have to be thankful. Amen.

Take some time to list the things you are thankful for this week. As you make your list, remember to keep it simple, keep it honest, keep it personal, and keep it specific.

When you think about what Jesus did for you—how He expressed His love for you on the cross—for what are you thankful?

When you think about the life He has called you to live, for what are you thankful?

As you look forward to what God will do in your heart and life through this study and your First Place 4 Health group, for what are you thankful?

"The best things are nearest: breath in your nostrils, light in your eyes, flowers at your feet, duties at your hand, the path of God just before you" (Robert Louis Stevenson).

Thank You, thank You, thank You, Lord, for each of these blessings and countless others that You have poured out on me. My heart is full of my love for You and Your love for me. Amen.

Notes

1. Ann Voskamp, *One Thousand Gifts: A Dare to Live Fully Right Where You Are* (Grand Rapids, MI: Zondervan, 2010), p. 15.
2. Carole Lewis, *A Thankful Heart: How Gratitude Brings Hope and Healing to Our Lives* (Ventura, CA: Regal Books, 2012), p.14.
3. Ibid, p. 16.
4. Ibid, p. 8.
5. Catherine Hart Weber, *Flourish: Discover the Daily Joy of Abundant, Vibrant Living* (Bloomington, MN: Bethany House, 2010), pp. 155-156.
6. Bill and Pam Farrel, *The Ten Best Decisions a Single Can Make* (Eugene, OR: Harvest House, 2011), p. 60.
7. For example, see the free app created for Ann Voskamp's *One Thousand Gifts*. You can add text and pictures to create your own list of a thousand things you're thankful for.
8. Lewis, *A Thankful Heart*, pp. 146-148.

Group Prayer Requests

4health first place

Today's Date: _____

Name	Request

Results

_____
_____
_____
_____
_____
_____

thankful for all things

SCRIPTURE MEMORY VERSE
*[Give] thanks to God the Father for everything,
in the name of our Lord Jesus Christ.*
EPHESIANS 5:20

Corrie ten Boom and her sister Betsie were Christians arrested for hiding Jews in their home during the Nazi occupation of Holland. They were sent to a concentration camp, where they experienced unspeakable suffering and torment. More than 1,400 sweat-soaked prisoners were crammed into barracks designed for 400. The plumbing backed up; the walls and floors were soiled and rancid. There were no individual cots, only rows of platforms to sleep on, precariously stacked three high and wedged side-by-side and end-to-end. The first night, the sisters discovered another horror: fleas! The place was swarming with them.

As they huddled together and prayed—asking God to show them how they could survive this place—Corrie and Betsie remembered the Scripture they had read that morning in a Bible they had managed to sneak past the guards during their check-in.

> "That's it, Corrie," Betsie said. "That's His answer. 'Give thanks in all circumstances.' That's what we can do. We can start right now to thank God for every single thing about this new barracks!"
>
> "Such as?" I [Corrie] said.
>
> "Such as being assigned here together."

I bit my lip. "Oh yes, Lord Jesus!"

"Such as what you're holding in your hands." I looked down at the Bible.

"Yes! Thank You, dear Lord, that there was no inspection when we entered here!"

"Thank you," Betsie went on serenely in prayer, "for the fleas and for . . ."

The fleas! This was too much. "Betsie, there's no way even God can make me grateful for a flea."

"Give thanks in all circumstances," she quoted. "It doesn't say 'in pleasant circumstances.' Fleas are part of this place where God has put us."

And so we stood between tiers of bunks and gave thanks for fleas. But this time I was sure Betsie was wrong.[1]

Corrie and Betsie began ministering to the other women in the barracks at night: comforting them, counseling them, leading them to Christ and discipling them in regular Bible studies and prayer meetings. For a while, they were afraid that at any moment, the guards might burst in and put a stop to it. But night after night they were able to minister uninterrupted. Later they found out that the guards refused to set foot in their barracks—because of the fleas!

How Corrie and Betsie's hearts overflowed with thanksgiving! And ours can too. We can give thanks for all things—even for fleas.

Day 1

GIVE THANKS

Lord Jesus, I'm in awe of Your amazing grace, of Your power made perfect in my weakness. Thank You for working in my heart and life. Amen.

Practice this week's memory verse by filling in the blanks below.

[Give] _____ to _____ the _____ for _____, in the _____ of our Lord _____ _____ (Ephesians 5:20).

Each day we have a choice to make. Will we trust God with whatever happens to us? Will we choose to believe that He is working all things for our good? Let's practice. Reread Romans 8:28 and make it personal. Fill in the blanks below with the things that are on your heart and mind.

"We know that in all things," even _____
"God works for the good of those who love him."

"We know that in all things," even _____
"God works for the good of those who love him."

"We know that in all things," even _____
"God works for the good of those who love him."

It's important to note that God doesn't call all things good, nor does He ask us to regard all things as such. Some things are ugly, hurtful, hateful and even downright evil—like a Nazi concentration camp. But God can take great evil and use it for greater good. (We'll explore this truth further in later chapters.)

So we always give thanks over all things, through all things and in the midst of all things, even *for* all things—because all things fit together into God's perfect plan. And one day, we will have the privilege of giving Him all the glory for it! As Betsie ten Boom told her sister Corrie:

> The most important part of our task will be to tell everyone who will listen that Jesus is the only answer to the problems that are disturbing the hearts of men and nations. We shall have the right to speak because we can tell from our experience that His light is more powerful than the deepest darkness. . . . How wonderful that the reality of His presence is greater than the reality of the hell about us![2]

Your circumstances may not be as horrific as those that the ten Boom sisters experienced, but undoubtedly you have faced some difficult, painful, even devastating circumstances of your own. In a few words, describe one such experience from your past.

What happened to your relationship with God during that troublesome time? Why?

Looking back, can you now see any good that came about as a result of the experience? If so, what?

Dear God, I choose to have a thankful heart. Teach me how to give thanks always, in everything, for Your glory! Amen.

Day 2

TO GOD THE FATHER

Father, I'm so thankful for Your love for me, thankful for Your protection and Your provision, Your constant care. Amen.

One of the reasons we can give thanks always, in everything, is because we know that nothing can come our way without first passing through the loving hands of our heavenly Father. We can't even begin to imagine all the hard or hurtful or even horrific things He stops—all the things He spares us from, the things He prevents from happening to us. When He does allow something painful or difficult or even tragic, we have His promise that there will be a purpose for it—a purpose in it—and His promise that He will be in it, too. What does God say to us in Isaiah 43:1-3?

What does Deuteronomy 31:8 tell us?

Look up Psalm 23 (even if you have it memorized). How does God care for us?

What don't we fear, and why (see verses 4-5)?

What does Deuteronomy 1:30-32 tell us?

Think of some of the troublesome times you have already come through. How was God with You? What did He do for you, in you and through you?

Father, I trust You with the challenges I face. Wrap me up in Your arms of love. Draw me close—so close I can hear Your heartbeat. Don't ever let me go. Amen.

Day 3 FOR EVERYTHING

Lord, teach me to be thankful for everything that comes my way. I know there's a blessing in each one somewhere! Amen.

English author G. K. Chesterton once remarked, "Jesus promised the disciples three things: that they would be completely fearless, absurdly happy and in constant trouble!" It's true. Jesus offers each of us an amazing adventure: a full life—full to overflowing! But what else did He tell us in John 16:33?

Why shouldn't we ever be discouraged?

If you were to travel to Israel and take a drive through the countryside, you would see that there are a lot of large, sprawling homes in the hills. You would probably conclude that the inhabitants must be quite wealthy. But then you might notice that the houses aren't as glamorous as they first appear. In fact, the different wings seem to be made of all different materials . . . almost as though they have been patched together, with additions built on and constructed at different times. If you asked a local guide, he or she would explain to you that it is a reflection of traditional Middle Eastern culture. From the moment a son is born into the family, the father begins setting aside building materials and supplies to add rooms in anticipation of the day that the son will bring home his bride. They will all live under one expanded roof together. What new insight does this give you into the meaning of Jesus' words in John 14:1-3?

Throughout the Scriptures, the marriage relationship between a husband and a wife is used as an analogy—an example or illustration—of the kind of loving, committed relationship God longs to have with each one of us individually and with humanity as a whole. He designed marriage for that very purpose. In the New Testament, the Church—which is made up of individual believers—is referred to collectively as "the Bride" (see, for example, Revelation 19:7). Jesus is pictured as the passionate Bridegroom who would do anything—even lay down His life—for His one true love (see, for example, Mark 2:19). Let's look at the traditional wedding vows that brides and grooms have been pledging since at least the early 1500s:

> **Groom:** I, [groom's name], take thee, [bride's name], to be my lawful wedded wife, to have and to hold from this day forward, for better for worse, for richer for poorer, in sickness and in health, to love and to cherish, till death us do part, according to God's holy ordinance; and thereto I plight thee my troth.

> **Bride:** I, [bride's name], take thee, [husband's name], to be my lawful wedded husband, to have and to hold from this day forward, for better for worse, for richer for poorer, in sickness and in health, to love, cherish, and to obey, till death us do part, according to God's holy ordinance; and thereto I give thee my troth.

How might these same vows apply to our relationship with our heavenly Bridegroom?

_____

_____

_____

_____

How does Christ keep His vows to us? How might we make—and keep—our vows to Christ?

_____

_____

_____

_____

Jesus, I give You my heart and my life. You are always faithful to me. Help me to be faithful always to You. Amen.

Day 4

IN THE NAME OF OUR LORD JESUS CHRIST

Lord, I thank You for each day, each opportunity You give me to live and love and learn, to grow deeper and draw closer to You. Amen.

Practice this week's verse by writing it (and the Scripture reference) from memory.

_____

_____

_____

_____

What does doing something "in the name of our Lord Jesus Christ" mean?

_____

_____

_____

_____

What does Acts 4:12 tell us about the name of Jesus?

_____

_____

_____

_____

Read Philippians 2:5-11. What name did God give Jesus (see verse 9)? One day, what will happen at the mention of the name of Jesus?

_____

_____

_____

Turn to 2 Thessalonians 1:11-12. What does Paul pray for believers living in the meantime, awaiting the Lord's return? Why?

_____

_____

_____

What does Titus 2:11-14 say about God's grace and what it teaches us, and what should we be doing while we wait for Jesus to come back?

_____

_____

_____

_____

What does Hebrews 13:15 urge us to do?

_____

_____

_____

Jesus, You are my Lord and Savior. How I long for Your return! Help me to make the most of this "meantime" and bring glory and honor to You. Amen.

TO THE GLORY OF GOD

Lord Jesus, I can never thank You enough for all that You have done for me.
Be glorified in my life. Amen.

The Bible teaches us that our vision—our perspective, our understanding—is limited. There is so much more going on than what we see, so much more taking place behind the scenes. There is so much more at stake in the choices that we make—more than we could ever imagine. Take a few minutes to read the first two chapters of the book of Job. What do we know that Job didn't know about his suffering (see Job 1:6-12; 2:1-6)?

_____

_____

_____

_____

What purpose did Job's suffering serve?

_____

_____

_____

_____

Even though he didn't see the big picture, didn't know the whole story, and couldn't have understood what was happening to him and why, how did Job respond (see Job 1:20-22; 2:10)?

_____

_____

_____

_____

When you read the book of Job, you find that Job did ask some honest questions. He debated the nature of suffering and the nature of God

Himself with those who came to comfort (really, to accuse) him. And eventually, God answered Job, though not the way Job expected. Turn to Job 42:10-17. What happened to Job in the latter part of his life?

_____

_____

_____

_____

In Psalm 40, David rejoiced that God had at last delivered him from his suffering. According to Psalm 40:3, what did God give him? What greater purpose did this serve?

_____

_____

_____

_____

How can you relate this to your life in general or to your journey with First Place 4 Health today?

_____

_____

_____

_____

Look at 2 Corinthians 4:15. As the number of believers in Christ grows, what also grows?

_____

_____

_____

_____

Lord, let me be a light shining for You in a dark and dying world.
May others see Your glory reflected in me and be drawn to You. Amen.

REFLECTION AND APPLICATION

*God, You are my strength and my shield—my song. My hope is in
You all day long. Amen.*

When disaster strikes, when tragedy occurs, or when things just go hor-
ribly wrong, how do you respond? What about when you're falsely accused, unjustly attacked or persecuted for taking a stand? (You *are*
taking a stand, aren't you?)

When troubles happen, we may be tempted to curl up in a ball and
cry a river of tears, throw ourselves a pity party or surrender to the feeling that we've been abandoned or forsaken by God. But that's not how
Paul and Silas responded when their stand resulted in horrible consequences (see Acts 16:16-40). Just for faithfully preaching the gospel,
these two men were severely beaten and thrown into prison, their feet
put in stocks. It would have been perfectly understandable if they'd
given in to discouragement and despair—if they'd laid there moaning
in pain or crying out to God in anguish.

But they didn't. The Bible tells us that at midnight, Paul and Silas
were praying and singing—but not a chorus of "Nobody Knows the
Trouble I've Seen." No, they were rejoicing and praising God, singing
hymns from their hearts to His. They were thanking Him for His goodness, mercy and love. Thanking Him. In prison.

God sent an earthquake to shake the prison walls, setting Paul and
Silas free. Because of their testimony in the midst of suffering and persecution, the jailor and all his household were saved. Sometimes the
most powerful praise comes from the darkest of times.

Few of us will ever be tortured and imprisoned like Paul and Silas,
but all of us have "dark nights of the soul"—times when discouragement
and despair threaten to overwhelm us. Moments when we wonder
what's going on and who's in control, and we wonder how we will survive. But no matter how difficult the battle, "we are more than con-
querors through him who loved us" (Romans 8:37): "Neither death nor
life, neither angels nor demons, neither our fears for today nor our wor-

ries about tomorrow—not even the powers of hell can separate us from God's love" (Romans 8:38, *NLT*).

The victory has been won. It's already ours. So we have every reason to rejoice, every reason to trust, every reason to give thanks—regardless of our circumstances. We know that God causes all things to work together "for the good of those who love him" (Romans 8:28). Let us remember the example of our brothers in Acts 16. If we offer up a sacrifice of praise, if we give thanks in all things, our eyes will be lifted from the misery of our circumstances to the beauty of our heavenly Father's face. We will find comfort and strength—and with our songs in the night, we will be a light to others.

Think about a particularly "dark" time in your life. Briefly describe what you went through and how you dealt with it. What part did God play?

Lord, thank You for the hardships, for the struggles, for the pain.
Be glorified in my life. In the name of Jesus, I pray. Amen.

REFLECTION AND APPLICATION

Day
7

Holy Spirit, bring to my remembrance all the things You have taught me
this week, and all the ways You have shown Your love for me. Amen.

Take some time to list the things you are thankful for this week. As you make your list, remember to keep it simple, keep it honest, keep it personal, and keep it specific.

In the space below, write a prayer thanking God for some of the hard times—the difficult and even painful things in your past—that He has already used for His glory and your good.

_____

_____

_____

_____

_____

Now write a prayer thanking God for some of the things that you are experiencing today, taking this opportunity to express your faith and trust in Him.

_____

_____

_____

_____

_____

Conclude by writing a prayer thanking God for the support He has given to you through your friends and your First Place 4 Health group.

_____

_____

_____

_____

_____

"God is in control, and therefore in everything [we] can give thanks—not because of the situation but because of the One who directs and rules over it" (Kay Arthur).

Thank You, thank You, thank You, Lord, for each of these blessings and countless others that You have poured out on me. My heart is full of my love for You and Your love for me. Amen.

Notes

1. Corrie ten Boom and John and Elizabeth Sherrill, *The Hiding Place* (Uhrichsville, OH: Barbour Publishing, 1971), pp. 209-210.
2. Corrie ten Boom, *Amazing Love: True Stories of the Power of Forgiveness* (Fort Washington, PA: CLC Publications, 2011), pp. 6-7.

Group Prayer Requests

4 first place health

Today's Date: _____

Name	Request

Results

_____
_____
_____
_____
_____

thankful for His blessings

SCRIPTURE MEMORY VERSE
Praise the LORD, O my soul, and forget not all his benefits.
PSALM 103:2

Years ago, a young woman shared that she had been going through a dark time in her life—a time when she was in so much physical, emotional and spiritual pain that she didn't want to be alive. She knew she couldn't kill herself, but she wished God would take her life. In fact, she prayed that He would! It just hurt too much to go on living.

One of her friends tried to help her see that things weren't as dark as they seemed and that there were brighter days ahead, but she wasn't convinced. She wanted hope; she just couldn't find any. The suffering she was experiencing might have been meant to produce character, but she didn't see herself becoming any more Christlike. She couldn't stand the thought of even one more trial and tribulation coming her way.

One day, after another long heart-to-heart talk, her friend made the young woman promise that for a month, before she went to bed every night, she would write down in a journal at least one blessing—one thing for which she was thankful. After all, her friend said, the Bible tells us to pray continually and to give thanks in every circumstance (see 1 Thessalonians 5:17-18). It's like the words of that old hymn: "When upon life's billows you are tempest tossed, when you are discouraged, thinking all is lost, count your many blessings, name them one by one, and it will surprise you what the Lord hath done."[1]

The first few days, all the young woman could think to write down was "I can breathe," "I can see," "I can hear" . . . but to be honest, she wasn't all that thankful for any of those things. Eventually, she began writing things such as, "I have a roof over my head," "I have a bed to sleep on," "My car still works—at least for now." But that got old quick. Still, a promise was a promise.

Soon, the woman started looking for something—anything—good that happened during the day, no matter how tiny or insignificant, just so she'd have something to write down. "I found a parking space close to the mall when it was raining." "I got a card from a friend." "My favorite praise and worship song came on the radio."

Little items turned into bigger one. Words of encouragement God was speaking to her heart. Miracles. Answers to prayer. The pages of her journal began to fill up. Now that she was looking for blessings, she was finding them everywhere, all around her. In time her faith was strengthened and her hope was renewed. Her depression lifted.

So, here's a question for you today: "Are you ever burdened with a load of care? Does the cross seem heavy you are called to bear?" If so, "Count your blessings, name them one by one, and it will surprise you what the Lord hath done."[2]

Day 1 HE FORGIVES MY SIN

Lord Jesus, today I will not forget Your benefits—the blessings You have poured out on me. I will praise You and thank You for every one! Amen.

When we count our blessings, we have to start with the greatest blessing of all: our salvation. Without it, none of the other blessings mean anything. All by itself, it is enough reason to thank God every moment, every day. What does Psalm 103:12 tell us God has done with our sins?

According to Jeremiah 31:34, what does God promise (see also Psalm 103:3; Ephesians 1:7)?

_____

_____

_____

_____

_____

Look up Micah 7:16-19. What do we learn about God in verse 18?

_____

_____

_____

_____

According to verse 19, what does God do with our sins?

_____

_____

_____

_____

Turn to Isaiah 1:18. In this verse, what does God say He will do with our sins when we ask for forgiveness?

_____

_____

_____

_____

How did Jesus accomplish this? What did it cost Him?

_____

_____

_____

_____

_____

Hymn writer Horatio Spafford exclaimed:

> My sin, oh, the bliss of this glorious thought!
> My sin, not in part but the whole,
> Is nailed to the cross, and I bear it no more,
> Praise the Lord, praise the Lord, O my soul.[3]

Take a few moments to reflect on today's Scriptures. Confess any sin you have yet to repent of, and receive God's forgiveness. Then write your own expression of praise and thanksgiving from your heart to God's.

_____

_____

_____

_____

_____

Jesus, I can never thank You enough for dying on the cross and shedding Your blood to save me from my sins. Live in my heart and be Lord of my life. Amen.

Day 2

HE HEALS ALL MY DISEASES

Lord, thank You for Your healing touch in my heart, my mind, my body and my spirit. Amen.

Practice this week's memory verse by filling in the blanks below.

_____ the _____, O my _____, and _____ not all his _____ (Psalm 103:2).

Every morning we wake up, we have something to be thankful for—a new day, a fresh start, the opportunity to experience God's love and mercy and grace—and share it with others. Some of us are in great health—and we tend to take it for granted. Others are works in progress, on journeys to better health. God is using First Place 4 Health to help us do our part to take care of the bodies He's given us. Some of us have major health issues—even life-threatening illnesses. We may or may not experience healing this side of heaven. But one way or another, our relief, our deliverance, our ultimate healing *is* coming! How would you describe your physical health right now?

_____

_____

_____

_____

How would you describe your mental health?

_____

_____

_____

_____

How would you describe your emotional health?

_____

_____

_____

_____

How would you describe your spiritual health?

_____

_____

_____

_____

Look up Psalm 30:2. What was the psalmist's testimony?

_____

_____

_____

_____

Look at 2 Corinthians 4:17-18. What blessings are there in suffering?

_____
_____
_____
_____
_____

Why should any type of disease or illness not cause us to lose hope?

_____
_____
_____
_____

If you have been healed, thank God! If you're in the process of being healed, thank Him! If you're holding on to the hope of heaven—and your ultimate healing—thank Him! Every single day.

> *Lord God, You are my Healer, my Helper and my Deliverer. Help me to honor You with the life You've given me. Amen.*

Day 3 — HE REDEEMS MY LIFE

Lord, thank You for Your amazing grace, Your unending mercy and Your redeeming love. Amen.

Look up Colossians 1:9-13. What did Paul pray for the believers in Colossae? What should we pray for ourselves and for each other (see verse 9)? Why is this so important?

_____
_____
_____
_____

Finish the following phrases from verses 10-12:

That you may _____

and may _____ :

bearing _____ ,

growing _____ ,

being _____

so that you may have _____ ,

and joyfully _____ .

What glorious truth do verses 13-14 proclaim?

_____

_____

_____

The *Life Application Study Bible, NIV* makes this observation concerning verse 13:

> True believers have been transferred from darkness to light, from slavery to freedom, from guilt to forgiveness, and from the power of Satan to the power of God. We have been rescued from a rebel kingdom to serve the rightful king.[4]

Talk about a reason to rejoice—a reason to give thanks! According to 1 Peter 1:18-19, how did God rescue us? How did He redeem us?

_____

_____

_____

Why was Jesus the only One who could redeem us (see verse 19)?

_____

_____

_____

What promise does God give His people in Joel 2:25?

_____

_____

_____

_____

In God's economy, nothing is wasted. He uses everything that happens to us, everything we experience—even our failures and mistakes—for our good and His glory. He redeems it all. Thank Him for that today.

Jesus, thank You for coming to my rescue, redeeming my life, restoring me to a right relationship with You. I bless You and praise Your holy name. Amen.

Day 4 — HE CROWNS ME WITH LOVE

Lord, I am Yours and You are mine. May my love for You abound more and more. Amen.

Our eternal blessings are the things we can forever thank God for. Look up 1 John 3:1. According to this verse, what is so wonderful, so great?

_____

_____

_____

_____

Turn to 1 John 4:9. How did God show His love for us?

_____

_____

_____

_____

Read Paul's prayer for believers in Ephesians 3:14-19. What two things did he pray first (see verses 16-17)?

_____

_____

_____

_____

Once God's Spirit is at work in us, once Christ dwells in our hearts through faith, once we've been rooted and established in love, what does Paul ask God to give us the power to grasp (see verse 18)?

_____

_____

_____

When we know this love—really know it, believe it, receive it and experience it for ourselves—what will happen to us (see verse 19)?

_____

_____

_____

_____

In other words, we'll have an experiential knowledge of God that is far greater, far deeper and far richer than we have now. Our hearts will be full to overflowing! Now read 2 Corinthians 1:3-4. How do these verses describe God?

_____

_____

_____

_____

When we know God in this way, what are we empowered to do?

_____

_____

_____

_____

> *God, thank You for Your love, Your compassion, Your mercy and grace.*
> *Thank You for Your comfort and peace. Help me to share all of these things*
> *with the people You send my way. Amen.*

Day 5

HE SATISFIES MY DESIRES

Lord, I can't thank You enough for Your many blessings and
Your love and faithfulness to me. Amen.

Look up Psalm 84. According to verses 1-2, what does the psalmist long for, or desire?

_____

_____

_____

_____

What does he declare in verse 10? Describe this in your own words.

_____

_____

_____

_____

_____

What promise do we find in verses 11-12?

_____

_____

_____

_____

When we trust God and His love for us, we trust Him not only to meet our needs but also to satisfy our desires—our good, Christ-honoring desires. These are the dreams and desires He Himself has put in our hearts. Can you think of some dreams or desires that God has given you? Which ones have been fulfilled?

_____

_____

_____

_____

_____

Which ones are still awaiting fulfillment?

_____

_____

_____

_____

What does Hebrews 10:23 urge us to do? Why?

_____

_____

_____

_____

How does Paul describe God in Ephesians 3:20?

_____

_____

_____

_____

Jesus, You know my heart's greatest longings, and You know how to fulfill them—for Your glory and my good. I entrust them to You. Amen.

REFLECTION AND APPLICATION

*Lord, may the words of my mouth and the meditation of my heart always
be pleasing to You. Amen (see Psalm 19:14).*

When we forget to count our blessings—when we focus on our disappointments and frustrations—we become negative, cranky, crabby people!

You know, being crabby all the time isn't just a shame, it's a sin! Whining, grumbling and complaining—when you get right down to it, these are symptoms of a selfish, ungrateful heart. A heart that wants its own way in everything—immediately—or else! Even God, who has infinite patience, can only take so much of it. The Old Testament tells us that the grumbling of the children of Israel very nearly drove Him to distraction—or at least to destruction, if Moses hadn't intervened—on more than one occasion. Their complaining revealed such a lack of faith and trust in God—in His leadership, His guidance, His provision, His power, His love. To God it was an insulting assault on His character (see Numbers 14:20-34).

That's no less true today. If we believe that God is in control of our circumstances, that whatever comes our way has first come through His hand, there's no excuse for the attitude that leads to whiny words. If we recognize that we ourselves are frail, flawed human beings who often sin and frequently fail to live up to others' expectations, then we have no excuse for ripping into anyone else. We're commanded not to be like ungodly "grumblers and faultfinders" (Jude 16). Instead, we are to "do everything without complaining or arguing, so that [we] may become blameless and pure, children of God without fault in a crooked and depraved generation, in which [we] shine like stars in the universe" (Philippians 2:14-15).

Our words (which are a reflection of our hearts) are a witness to our friends, family, neighbors, co-workers and the entire world around us. Our words are a testimony of who God is and what His people are like. Around the house or the office, in the car or the classroom, at the grocery store or gas station, let's choose to let our light shine through the words that we speak: words of hope, trust, peace, patience and contentment; words of praise and thanksgiving. After all, God is good. And we are in His care.

How can what you do and say turn people away from God and discourage them from becoming believers?

_____

_____

_____

_____

_____

How can you act and speak in a way that attracts people to God and encourages them to want to choose to follow Christ?

_____

_____

_____

_____

Father, forgive me for the times I've tested Your patience with my grumbling and complaining. Fill my lips with Your praise. Help me to bring joy to Your heart today and every day! Amen.

REFLECTION AND APPLICATION

Day 7

Holy Spirit, please bring to my remembrance all the things that You have taught me this week, all the ways You have shown Your love for me, all the things for which I have to be thankful. Amen.

Take some time to list the things you are thankful for this week. As you make your list, remember to keep it simple, keep it honest, keep it personal, and keep it specific.

_____

_____

_____

_____

_____

In the space below, write a prayer thanking God for some of the spiritual blessings He has given you.

_____

_____

_____

_____

_____

_____

Now write a prayer thanking God for giving you people in your First Place 4 Health group who provide blessings to you.

_____

_____

_____

_____

_____

_____

Conclude by writing a prayer asking God for the grace and strength and courage you need to keep counting your blessings, one by one.

_____

_____

_____

_____

_____

_____

"Thou who hast given so much to me, give me one thing more: a grateful heart" (George Herbert).

Thank You, thank You, thank You, Lord, for each of these blessings and countless others that You have poured out on me. My heart is full of my love for You and Your love for me. Amen.

Notes

1. Ira D. Sankey, "Count Your Blessings," 1897.
2. Ibid.
3. Horatio Spafford, "It Is Well with My Soul," 1873.
4. Note on Colossians 1:13, *The Life Application Study Bible, NIV* (Carol Stream, IL: Tyndale House Publishers, 2005).

Group Prayer Requests

4 first place
health

Today's Date: _____

Name	Request

Results

_____

_____

_____

_____

_____

thankful
for our thorns

SCRIPTURE MEMORY VERSE
For Christ's sake, I delight in weaknesses, in insults, in hardships, in persecutions, in difficulties. For when I am weak, then I am strong.
2 CORINTHIANS 12:10

In 2 Corinthians 12:7-10, Paul talks about wrestling with "a thorn in [his] flesh"—a persistent problem, a constant struggle, a real battle—an area in which victory seemed impossible (verse 7). Paul says, "Three times I pleaded with the Lord to take it away from me. But he said to me, 'My grace is sufficient for you, for my power is made perfect in weakness'" (verses 8-9).

Many of us can relate. But even more of us can relate to the problem of a thorn in our side, which is a whole different thing—or, rather, a person. In Numbers 33:55 and Judges 2:3, God uses the phrase "thorns in your sides" to describe people who persistently trouble us, irritate us, frustrate us, mistreat us, distract us from our calling, and tempt us to fall into sin.

Every one of us has at least one "thorn," one difficult person in our lives. Maybe more than one! Think about it. When you hear the phrase "a thorn in my side"—whose name comes to mind? The Bible tells us that those people are the very ones God wants us to thank Him for. The very people He wants us to love unconditionally, no matter how unlovable they seem. Author Virelle Kidder observes:

Loving is the most important work any of us will ever do, and it's seldom easy. Only God's grace gives us the love for others we need, but it's the best reason there is to get up every morning. And the only way the world, and those we love, will ever know God is real.[1]

This week, we'll learn how to be thankful for the thorns in our sides and find hope and healing—for them and for us.

LOVING OUR THORNS

*Lord, teach me to love as You love. Give me a heart for the difficult people
You have placed in my life. Amen.*

Look up Matthew 22:36-40. What did Jesus say is the greatest commandment (see verses 37-38)?

_____

_____

_____

_____

_____

What is the second greatest commandment (see verse 39)?

_____

_____

_____

_____

_____

Now turn to Luke 6:27-36. To the shock and amazement of His listeners, Jesus added what four things (see verses 27-28)?

1. _____

2. _____

3. _____

4. _____

Why should we be merciful to difficult people (see verses 32-35)?

_____

_____

_____

_____

_____

As Jesus Himself pointed out, it's easy to love people who love you. But loving those people who irritate you, annoy you or offend you; loving people who hurt you or betray you—or hurt and betray people you love—now that takes a miracle! A miracle God wants to do in you and through you. He loves you. After all, He loved you when you were at your worst, most miserable, most unlovable. And He wants you to extend that love to others (see John 15:12). According to 1 John 4:20, what is the true test, the evidence, of whether or not we really love God and obey His commandments?

_____

_____

_____

_____

_____

God is serious about this. He really means it. He uses difficult people in our lives to teach us many things, including how to love as He loves. And until we learn what He wants us to learn, He will keep putting difficult people in our paths! However, as Carole Lewis says, "As we learn to thank God for the people who give us the most problems, we let go of the problems and allow God to begin working, not only in our life but in the life of the other person as well."[2]

Lord, do a work in my heart. I'm willing—or willing to be made willing—
to let You love the difficult people in my life through me. Amen.

LEARNING FROM OUR THORNS

*Father, thank You for Your grace, which is sufficient for me. Your power
is made perfect in my weakness (see 2 Corinthians 12:9). Amen.*

Practice this week's memory verse by filling in the blanks below.

For _____ sake, I _____ in _____, in _____, in
_____, in _____, in _____. For when I am
_____, then I am _____ (2 Corinthians 12:10).

Difficult people have so much to teach us—about God, about themselves,
about ourselves. Sometimes our conflicts come about as a result of dif-
ferences in our backgrounds, cultures and upbringings; or in our God-
given temperaments, personalities, gifts and talents; or in our approaches,
perspectives and attitudes. If we allow God to soften our hearts, we can
come to understand these people (at least a little) and respect or even appreciate who they are and what they bring to the table. According to
Ephesians 4:2, how should we approach all of our relationships?

_____

_____

_____

_____

Sometimes God uses difficult people to show us just how selfish, impatient, irritable and inflexible we can be; how quick we are to become angry, critical or judgmental; how much we have to learn, how much we
need to grow—if we want to be more like Jesus. We're reminded of how
much we need a Savior, because it turns out we're mixed-up, messed-up,
broken people just like our thorns! Look up Colossians 3:12-14. What
are we to clothe ourselves with (see verses 12)?

_____

_____

_____

How should we handle conflicts and disagreements (see verse 13)?

_____

_____

_____

_____

When we have trouble forgiving someone, what should we remember that will make our forgiveness easier to extend (see verse 13)?

_____

_____

_____

_____

What are we to put over our virtues to bind them together (see verse 14)?

_____

_____

_____

Difficult people give us the opportunity to put these principles into practice. Because of them, we get to practice becoming more godly, more mature, more Christlike—which is what we pray for, isn't it? We should thank them for that! Carole Lewis notes, "It has been my experience that after I've learned the lesson God has for me, He either heals the other person or He moves them on to some other place. In either case, I am better off as I learn to love the difficult people in my life."[3] What lessons have you learned so far by dealing with difficult people in your life?

_____

_____

_____

Father, You have been so kind, so loving, so gracious and so merciful to me. You did not treat me as my sins deserved. Help me to be kind, loving, gracious and merciful to others. Amen.

LIVING WITH OUR THORNS

Lord Jesus, please give me strength and patience and peace to deal with the difficult people in my life. Amen.

Someone once said, "Love your enemies—it'll drive them crazy!" Sometimes we may feel as if the difficult people in our lives are driving *us* crazy—especially when we have to spend time with them on a continual basis. Read 2 Corinthians 6:4-10. What kinds of difficult things does God call His servants to endure (see verses 4-5,8-10)?

_____

_____

_____

_____

_____

What character qualities, or attributes, does He call us to demonstrate (see verses 6-7)?

_____

_____

_____

_____

What weapons do we carry (see verse 7)?

_____

_____

_____

_____

Look at Romans 13:12,14. What sort of armor do we have?

_____

_____

_____

_____

Turn to 2 Corinthians 10:3-5. What do our weapons have the power to do?

_____

_____

_____

_____

Read Ephesians 6:10-18. What is the full armor of God (see verses 13-18)?

_____

_____

_____

_____

Why do we need God's mighty power? Who or what do we fight (see verses 11-12)?

_____

_____

_____

_____

The mention of weapons reminds us there are times when we absolutely need to stand up and fight for righteousness as we live with our thorns. Sometimes we have to establish clear, Biblical boundaries in our difficult relationships. If you need help in this area, talk to a trusted friend, a pastor or a Christian counselor; or pick up a book such as Leslie Vernick's *The Emotionally Destructive Relationship: Seeing It, Stopping It, Surviving It.* We have to take responsibility for our part in all of our relationships—even particularly thorny ones—making sure that our behavior is Christ-honoring and above reproach. What admonition do we find in Romans 12:17-18?

_____

_____

_____

_____

These verses tell us not to respond to bad behavior with bad behavior of our own, not to seek vengeance on our own. Sometimes conflict can't be avoided. We can't control how others respond. There are problems that have to be addressed—directly, appropriately, respectfully, authoritatively—but not vengefully. Ultimately it's God's responsibility to settle the score—He is the righteous judge (see Romans 12:19).

God, give me the wisdom to respond to difficult people biblically, courageously and lovingly. In Jesus' name I pray. Amen.

Day 4

FORGIVING OUR THORNS

Holy Spirit, shine the light of truth in my heart and help me to hear what You have to say to me. Amen.

Brace yourself for a challenging truth and a painful reality: you are a difficult person. Yes, *you.* You get on people's nerves, irritate them and annoy them. Sometimes, you hurt them, mistreat them, misunderstand them and misjudge them. Sorry to say it, but despite your best efforts, you aren't always polite, thoughtful, loving and kind. There are things about your personality and temperament that make you difficult to get along with, work with or live with—at least for some people. You just rub them the wrong way, even when you don't mean to do it (and sometimes you *do* mean to do it). Somewhere in the world today, someone is praying that God will give them the grace to love and forgive you. How does Luke 6:31 tell us we should treat others?

Read the following statements and check all that apply:

_____ I want to be heard.

_____ I want to be respected.

_____ I want to be understood.

_____ I want to be loved.

_____ I want others to be kind to me.

_____ I want others to be merciful to me.

_____ I want others to be considerate of me.

_____ I want others to refrain from judging me.

_____ I want others to refrain from criticizing me.

_____ I want others to refrain from gossiping about me.

_____ I want others to refrain from complaining about me.

_____ I want others to give me the benefit of the doubt.

_____ I want others to forgive me.

There you go. This is how you should treat others! What stern warning do we find in Matthew 7:1-2?

_____

_____

_____

_____

If you really believed this—if you took it to heart—how would it affect the way you judge the difficult people in your life today?

_____

_____

_____

_____

What other warning do we find in Matthew 6:14-15?

_____

_____

_____

_____

_____

Look at Ephesians 4:32. Since we want to be more Christlike, why should we forgive others?

_____

_____

_____

_____

_____

In our flesh, it may seem impossible to love and forgive difficult people. But God can. After all, He loves and forgives us! And He will love and forgive through us, if we ask Him.

> _Lord Jesus, help me to obey Your Word. Help me to love. Help me to forgive. Help me to treat others the way I want to be treated. Amen._

Day 5

PRAYING FOR OUR THORNS

Lord, I lift up my "thorns" to You and ask You to meet them where they are—and draw them closer to You. Amen.

Look at Matthew 5:44. What did Jesus tell us to do?

_____

_____

_____

_____

We've got to resist the urge to pray that God will "deal" with the person—that He will judge them or punish them or "fix" them. That kind of prayer all too quickly turns into a rehearsal of our grievances: We start making our case against the other person, while declaring our own innocence. This is not what Jesus asked us to do. Instead, we need to thank God for bringing these people into our lives. We need to ask Him to teach us what He wants us to learn—about Him, about them, about us. We need to ask Him to help us to see these people as He sees them and to love them with His love. We need to pray for the difficult people in our lives the same way we pray for ourselves—the way we pray for our friends and families, the way we want them to pray for us. Look up each of the following verses and list the things you can pray for others today:

Ephesians 1:16: _____

Ephesians 1:17: _____

Ephesians 1:18-19: _____

Ephesians 3:16-17: _____

Ephesians 3:17-19: _____

Colossians 1:9: _____

Colossians 1:10: _____

Colossians 1:11: _____

If the difficult people in your life don't already know Jesus, then that's the first place to start: Pray that they will come to a saving knowledge of Him. As you pray for these people, you will discover an amazing truth: God can completely change your heart! He can fill you with His love for the most unlikely, most unlovable people. He can love them and draw them to Himself through you.

Lord, help me to be faithful in prayer—even for my enemies and for other difficult people I find so hard to love. I may well be the only person praying for them. Then again, there may be many of us storming heaven on their behalf. Either way, I want to do my part, just as You've asked. Amen.

REFLECTION AND APPLICATION

*Lord, thank You for the people who loved me, even when I was unlovable.
Help me to love others and lead them to You. Amen.*

Are you a Pollyanna? Today the word "Pollyanna" is often used as a derogatory term to describe a person who is naively optimistic, intentionally blind to unpleasant truths, or willfully and woefully out of touch with the harsh realities of life. But if you've ever read the original novel written by Eleanor H. Porter or seen the Disney movie featuring Hayley Mills, then you know better.

Pollyanna is a little girl whose minister-father taught her from a very early age to cultivate in her heart "an attitude of gratitude." Together, father and daughter play "the glad game," in which they try to help each other find something to be glad about or grateful for in every situation, no matter how difficult or unpleasant it may at first seem. In other words, in every cloud, they look for a silver lining. Pollyanna's father also teaches his daughter an important lesson that he confesses he had to learn the hard way: Always look for the good in others, rather than focus on their faults and flaws. It's something that has helped him become a better pastor and person.

As the story unfolds, the young girl experiences more than her fair share of heartache. Both of her beloved parents die, and she's sent to live with a wealthy aunt she's never met before. The aunt is a cold and distant woman who dominates the social structure of an unhappy and unfriendly town. But even in this unwelcoming environment, surrounded by negative, complaining, miserable people, Pollyanna proves that her spirit cannot be stifled or subdued.

Just as her father taught her, Pollyanna looks for the good in everyone and everything—and she finds it! She brings out the best in the crabbiest, crankiest, most difficult people. Her enthusiasm is so contagious that it spreads from one person to another and another. Even her hardhearted aunt can't help but soften in response to Pollyanna's steadfast determination to rejoice and be glad.

In the end, when Pollyanna faces a loss that for the first time threatens to overwhelm even her resolutely cheerful spirit, the townspeople rally around her. One by one they share with her how she has made a difference in their lives. They repeat to her the very words she once said to them—words of love and friendship, hope and faith. They repeat words that have come from a happy heart, a thankful heart.

We all could learn a thing or two from Pollyanna. There are so many lost and sin-sick souls, so many desperate and hurting (and yes, difficult) people in the world. We can be a light in the darkness by choosing to have happy hearts, thankful hearts; by choosing to look for the good in those around us and encouraging them to do the same. Why not be a Pollyanna in someone else's life today![4]

In what ways might you be able to be a Pollyanna to someone you know?

_____

_____

_____

Jesus, let my thankful heart and my love for You shine through in everything I say and do. May others be drawn to You, too. Amen.

REFLECTION AND APPLICATION

Day 7

Holy Spirit, please bring to my remembrance all the things that You have taught me this week, all the ways You have shown Your love for me, all the things for which I have to be thankful. Amen.

Take some time to list the things you are thankful for this week. As you make your list, remember to keep it simple, keep it honest, keep it personal and keep it specific.

_____

_____

_____

_____

In the space below, write a prayer thanking God for forgiving you—for not holding your sins against you today.

_____

_____

_____

_____

_____

_____

Write a prayer thanking God for giving you grace to forgive your "thorns." Thank Him for making you willing—or willing to be made willing.

_____

_____

_____

_____

Conclude by writing a prayer thanking God for the opportunity to be a positive influence in the lives of those in your First Place 4 Health group. Think of specific ways you can have an impact on them today.

_____

_____

_____

_____

_____

_____

"The optimist says the cup is half full. The pessimist says the cup is half empty. The child of God says, 'My cup runneth over'" (Anonymous).

Thank You, thank You, thank You, Lord, for each of these blessings and countless others that You have poured out on me. My heart is full of my love for You and Your love for me. Amen.

Notes

1. Virelle Kidder, *The Best Life Ain't Easy, But It's Worth It* (Chicago: Moody Publishers, 2008), p. 99.
2. Carole Lewis, *A Thankful Heart: How Gratitude Brings Hope and Healing to Our Lives* (Ventura, CA: Regal Books, 2012), p. 37.
3. Ibid.
4. Christin Ditchfield, *A Way with Words: What Women Should Know About the Power They Possess* (Wheaton, IL: Crossway Books, 2010), pp. 61-62.

Group Prayer Requests

4 first place
health

Today's Date: _____

Name	Request

Results

_____

_____

_____

_____

_____

thankful
for His provision

SCRIPTURE MEMORY VERSE

[Do not] put [your] hope in wealth, which is so uncertain, but . . . put [your] hope in God, who richly provides us with everything for our enjoyment.

1 TIMOTHY 6:17

Maybe you've seen the old cartoon that features a puzzled young woman talking to a bank manager. She asks, "How can I be out of money? I still have checks!" Balancing the checkbook, juggling the bills—these days it's not easy to make ends meet. Some of us are pinching pennies until they squeal! We don't know how we're going to make it to the end of the month. And it's not just money. We're pressed for time, for energy and for answers to our family problems or to crises at work.

The good news is that even when our resources run low—or run out—we have somewhere to turn. We need only to ask our heavenly Father for what we need: wisdom to make good choices; strength to resist temptation; peace to calm our fears. In Psalm 50:10, He reminds us that He owns the cattle on a thousand hills. He also owns the hills! And every blade of grass on those hills—and the sun that warms them! The universe and everything in it belongs to Him. His resources are endless. He owns it all. And out of His great love and kindness, our Father generously provides for us, His children. What's His is ours.

Philippians 4:19 tells us, "God will meet all your needs according to his glorious riches in Christ Jesus." He provides for our physical needs and our spiritual needs. Sometimes He miraculously provides what we need: money in an unmarked envelope, groceries on the doorstep, a cancelled meeting that opens up some precious time in our schedule. Suddenly, we have the creative inspiration or the problem-solving solution we've been searching for. Seemingly from nowhere we are given the wisdom, the encouragement, the direction and the victory. Sometimes, He shows us how to make better use of the resources He's already given us. And sometimes, He helps us see the difference between what we really *want* and what we truly *need*. But no matter what, our Father never abandons us, never forsakes us. He always answers when we call.

Whenever you feel your resources are stretched to their limits, turn to the One whose supplies are limitless. He promises to meet your every need—and that's something you can be thankful for every day!

THE GIFT

Lord, I'm so grateful for Your faithful provision. You have promised to meet all of my needs, and I take You at Your word. Amen.

Fill in the blanks below to complete this week's Scripture memory verse.

[Do not] _____ [your] _____ in _____, which is so _____, but _____ [your] _____ in _____, who richly _____ us with _____ for our _____ (1 Timothy 6:17).

Our goal this week is to learn to have a thankful heart, regardless of our financial circumstances or other needs—and to trust in God's promises to provide for us. As John MacArthur observes:

A thankful heart is one of the primary identifying characteristics of a believer. It stands in stark contrast to pride, selfishness, and worry. And it helps fortify the believer's trust in the Lord and reliance of His provision, even in the toughest times. No matter how choppy the seas become, a believer's heart is buoyed by constant praise and gratefulness to the Lord.

Let's look at how Jesus provided for the needs of those He encountered in His earthly ministry. Read each of the passages in the chart below and then identify the need that is described and how it was met.

Matt. 14:15-21	Need (see verses 15-17):	Provision (see verses 18-21):
Matt. 17:24-27	Need (see verse 24):	Provision (see verse 27):
Mark 5:25-34	Need (see verse 26):	Provision (see verses 29,34):
Mark 9:17-27	Obvious need (see verses 17-18,21-22): Deeper need (see verse 24):	Provision (see verse 27):

Carole Lewis states, "In my own life, financial problems [a failed business and a bankruptcy] were the tools God used to bring me to the end of myself so that He could remake me into the woman He had always wanted me to be. I am forever grateful for our money woes, because they were the vehicle that drove me to God."[1] Read Psalm 107, which describes four types of people whose needs God fulfills. The first group is described as those who are lost (verses 4-9). What does God do for them (see verses 7,9)?

_____

_____

_____

_____

The members of the second group are described as prisoners (verse 10). How does God rescue them (see verses 14,16)?

_____

_____

_____

The third group is made up of those who have brought about their own problems (verse 17). How does God fulfill their needs (see verse 20)?

_____

_____

_____

In the fourth group are those who suffer storms at sea (though this could also apply to the storms of life). What does God do to provide for them (see verses 29-30)?

_____

_____

_____

Jesus, search my heart. See my needs. Meet each one according to Your will, according to Your plans and purposes for me. Amen.

Day 2 — THE CHOICE

Thank You, Lord, for each new day, each new opportunity to trust and hope in You. Amen.

The disciples asked Jesus to teach them how to pray. He gave them a prayer that we can pray just as He did *and* use as a model for our own prayers. Read the Lord's Prayer in Matthew 6:9-13. For what should we ask God?

_____

_____

_____

Read Matthew 6:19-21. Jesus describes a choice we have about what sort of treasure we can store up for ourselves. What specific "treasures on earth" are you storing up? On what does your heart focus?

_____

_____

_____

_____

What specifically could you do to instead store up treasures in heaven?

_____

_____

_____

_____

Read Matthew 6:25-34. What does Jesus tell us _not_ to worry about (see verse 25)? What reasons does Jesus give for why we shouldn't worry?

_____

_____

_____

_____

Instead of worrying, what should we choose to do (see verse 33)?

_____

_____

_____

_____

_____

In what practical ways could you show what you have chosen to seek?

_____

_____

_____

_____

What does God promise (see verse 33)?

_____

_____

_____

Lord, help me to seek first Your kingdom—to give You first place in
my heart and life today and every day. Amen.

THE SECRET

Father, I bring You all the things that worry me or concern me—and I
leave them in Your far-more-capable hands. Amen.

God uses our times of need to draw us closer to Him, to teach us to look
to Him and lean on Him and depend on Him each day. He teaches us
that ultimately He is our provider, and that in the end, He is really all we
need. Look up Philippians 4:11-13. What does Paul say he has learned
(see verses 11-12)?

_____

_____

_____

In what different kinds of circumstances did Paul find himself (see verse
12; see also 2 Corinthians 11:24-28)?

_____

_____

_____

Paul's experiences gave him the authority to speak on the subject, and we
can trust what he has to say on it. So what does Paul say is the key—the
secret—to contentment (see Philippians 4:13)?

_____

_____

_____

Of what three things does Paul remind us in 1 Timothy 6:6-8?

1. _____

2. _____

3. _____

What does 2 Peter 1:3 assure us?

_____

_____

_____

What encouragement do we find in 2 Corinthians 9:8?

_____

_____

_____

Lord, help me take to heart the secret of being content. Help me in everything I say and do to bring glory and honor to You. Amen.

THE BATTLE Day 4

Jesus, guard my heart and mind. Keep me from trusting in anything or anyone but You. Amen.

During His earthly ministry, Jesus had a lot to say about money—perhaps because it is such a preoccupation, such a distraction, and such a temptation for nearly all of us. No matter how much or how little we have, we're tempted to think that more would be better! More money would solve all of our problems, make us safe and secure, and give us peace of mind. All too easily, money can become an idol. Look at Luke 16:13. What warning did Jesus give us?

_____

_____

_____

Read the parable of the sower in Mark 4:1-20. What "weeds" choked the Word of God and kept it from bearing fruit (see verses 18-19)?

_____

_____

_____

Scottish missionary David Livingstone once said, "Do not think me mad. It is not to make money that I believe a Christian should live. The noblest thing a man can do is, just humbly to receive, and then go amongst others and give." Read 1 Timothy 6:9-10. What happens to people who make it their goal—their life's mission—to accumulate wealth (see verse 9)?

_____

_____

_____

You've probably heard the expression, a misquote of 1 Timothy 6:10: "Money is the root of all evil." What does the verse actually say?

_____

_____

_____

According to this verse, what is the most tragic consequence of making money your true love?

_____

_____

_____

Look up 1 Timothy 6:17-19, the passage in which this week's memory verse appears. What should those blessed with financial resources hope in (see verse 17)?

_____

_____

_____

How should they live (see verse 18)? What purpose will this serve (see verse 19)?

_____

_____

_____

*Lord Jesus, help me to honor You with my finances—and all of
my resources—today and every day. May they have their proper place in
my life, and may they be used only for Your glory. Amen.*

THE BLESSING

Day
5

*Lord, I realize that everything I am, and everything I have is a gift from You.
I give it back to You now, to be used for Your kingdom and Your glory. Amen.*

Look up Romans 12:4-8. Of all the spiritual gifts mentioned, which one is related to our theme this week (see verse 8)?

_____

_____

_____

Not everybody has the gift of giving, but everyone can give. Turn to Mark 12:41-44. What did Jesus say about the significance—and the size—of the widow's gift?

_____

_____

_____

Martin Luther once observed, "The heart of the giver makes the gift dear and precious." Look up 2 Corinthians 9:7. What does God want us to give, and how should we give?

_____

_____

_____

Read Romans 12:13. Who does God want us to give to?

_____

_____

_____

Turn to Acts 20:35. What did Jesus tell us about giving?

_____

_____

_____

_____

What does Proverbs 11:25 say?

_____

_____

_____

Read 2 Corinthians 9:10-11. Why does God bless us?

_____

_____

_____

_____

God, thank You for the time and energy, the gifts and talents, and the financial resources You have given me. Help me to give freely, cheerfully, generously, as You lead me today and every day. Amen.

Day 6 — REFLECTION AND APPLICATION

Lord Jesus, open my heart to receive all that You have for me. Amen.

As the children of Israel began their wilderness wanderings, they grumbled and complained that God had brought them out of slavery in Egypt only to let them starve in the desert. God, in His mercy, provided for them by sending manna—bread from heaven. This miraculous food was like nothing they had ever seen (which is why they called it manna—meaning "what is it?"). Every day it appeared on the ground like the dew. "Each morning everyone gathered as much as he needed," and they had enough to eat (Exodus 16:21).

There was one other thing about the manna that was unusual: It didn't keep. The Israelites couldn't store it up and save it for a rainy day. They had to gather a fresh supply every morning. They had to look to God for His provision each new day.

Those of us who have been Christians for some time will have had many experiences in the past where we saw God work in our lives. But if we're not careful, we can find ourselves leaning a little too heavily on the "glory days" gone by. We can be content to simply regurgitate stuff we learned years ago when our heavenly Father has so much more to teach us, so much more to say. But there's no need to chew on stale bread. God has a fresh Word to give us each day.

In Psalm 81:10, God says, "I am the LORD your God, who brought you up out of Egypt. Open wide your mouth and I will fill it." All we have to do is receive God's provision. Take time now to quiet your heart before the Lord. He has something new to say to you today! Read His Word, talk to Him in prayer—and listen. What is God saying to you today?

What do you want to say to God?

Thank You, Lord, for providing everything I need, moment by moment, day by day. You are so faithful, Lord! Amen.

REFLECTION AND APPLICATION

Holy Spirit, please bring to my remembrance all the things that You have taught me this week, all the ways You have shown Your love for me, all the things for which I have to be thankful. Amen.

Take some time to list the things you are thankful for this week. As you make your list, remember to keep it simple, keep it honest, keep it personal, and keep it specific.

_____

_____

_____

_____

_____

In the space below, write a prayer thanking God for His provision today—His provision for you financially, physically, emotionally, and spiritually.

_____

_____

_____

_____

_____

Write a prayer thanking God for providing for your future needs—those needs you anticipate, and those you can't.

_____

_____

_____

_____

_____

Conclude by writing a prayer to thank Him for the things He has given to you to give to others (such as your time, your talents and your resources.) Think about someone in your First Place 4 Health group with whom you could share, and ask God to help you share these things fully and freely as He leads.

_____

_____

_____

_____

_____

> The discipline of gratitude is the explicit effort to acknowledge that all I am and have is given to me as a gift of love, a gift to be celebrated with joy (Henri J. M. Nouwen).

Thank You, thank You, thank You, Lord, for each of these blessings and countless others that You have poured out on me. My heart is full of my love for You and Your love for me. Amen.

Note

1. Carole Lewis, *A Thankful Heart: How Gratitude Brings Hope and Healing to Our Lives* (Ventura, CA: Regal Books, 2012), p. 44.

Group Prayer Requests

first place
4health

Today's Date: _____

Name	Request

Results

_____

_____

_____

_____

_____

_____

thankful
for His plan

SCRIPTURE MEMORY VERSE

Show me your ways, O LORD, teach me your paths; guide me in your truth and teach me, for you are God my Savior, and my hope is in you all day long.

PSALM 25:4-5

Growing up, Amy really didn't like the color of her eyes. She thought of them as dull and ordinary—a plain old brown—while her sister's eyes were such a beautiful blue! Amy attended church regularly with her family. During one service, she heard a powerful guest preacher say that God can do anything, and that if we really believe in our hearts and ask Him to do something, He will. So that night at bedtime, Amy prayed as hard as she knew how that God would turn her brown eyes blue.

The next morning, she ran to the bathroom to look in the mirror, confident her request had been heard and answered. Well, it had—but not the way she wanted. God had said no. He didn't change the color of Amy's eyes. He left them the color He had made them. For a while, Amy was heartbroken. She didn't understand. She *couldn't* understand . . . at least, not yet.

But many years later, God called Amy Carmichael to become a missionary to India. Amy found that when she dressed in traditional Indian clothing, with her skin stained dark with tea leaves and brown eyes, she didn't stand out like a typical European tourist. She blended in with the other women of the community. This made it possible for Amy to slip in and out of Hindu temples unnoticed—and rescue hundreds of little girls who had been sold into slavery and prostitution.

As Amy discovered, her brown eyes weren't a random act of genetics or a sign she was any less loved or favored by God. They were, in fact, a precious gift from God to help her accomplish His unique plan and purpose for her life. No wonder He wouldn't change them!

God tells us that we are His workmanship, His creation, His masterpiece! Over and over, the Scriptures say that God made each one of us the way we are for a reason. Before we were even born, He had a plan and a purpose for our lives—a specific calling and a certain path He had chosen for us. He has kingdom work for us to do!

We may not always appreciate this powerful truth. Often, we will have our own ideas of how we should look or what we should be like. We may think we would be happier if we had someone else's appearance or personality or gifts. But God knows us best. After all, He created us, and, lest we forget, *He* is the potter; we are the clay (see Isaiah 64:8, Jeremiah 18:1-6.) God molds us and shapes us as He sees fit, and He is able to work even with our missteps and mistakes and turn our weakness into strength. We can trust Him, even when we don't understand.[1]

Day 1 · SOVEREIGN LORD

Lord, I thank You that You have a plan and a purpose for me. You know what is best and You do what is best. All the time, You are good. Amen.

Practice this week's memory verse by filling in the blanks below.

_____ me your _____, O Lord, _____ me your _____; guide me in your _____ and _____ me, for you are _____ my _____, and my _____ is in _____ all _____ long (Psalm 25:4-5).

Look up Ephesians 1:11-12. Of what are we a part? What is it that makes our lives meaningful?

_____

_____

_____

Turn to Psalm 71:15-16. How does the psalmist address God?

_____

_____

_____

_____

This name for God appears nearly 300 times in the Old and New Testaments! The word "sovereign" means having supreme, unlimited power or authority—complete control. To be sovereign is to be preeminent; indisputable; greatest in degree; utmost or extreme; above all others in character, importance and excellence. Although God is sovereign over our lives, we don't always acknowledge Him as being the most important in our lives. What are some of the things of this world that too often compete for our attention and draw it away from our Sovereign Lord?

_____

_____

_____

_____

Look up Colossians 1:15-18. What do these verses tell us about Jesus?

_____

_____

_____

When we looked at Romans 8:28 earlier in this study, we learned that God uses His authority and power to work out for our good everything that happens. Even though we live in a fallen world and evil exists, God can and does use all of what we experience for our good. What things do you need to trust God to work together for good in your life today?

_____

_____

_____

_____

How can your First Place 4 Health group help you as you seek to trust God's sovereignty?

_____

_____

_____

_____

As author, preacher and Bible teacher, John Piper points out, God was able to take the most "spectacular" sin (the greatest evil, the most wicked injustice) in the history of the world—the crucifixion of Jesus—and use it to triumph over the devil, redeem His children and glorify His Son.[2] Trust Him to work in your heart and life today.

> *Lord, I bring You everything that is on my heart today, everything that troubles me or frustrates me or worries me. I surrender them to You and ask You to do Your will in each of these things, for Your glory and my good. Amen.*

Day 2

THE MASTER'S PLAN

Lord, before I was born, You had a plan and a purpose for me. Help me to fulfill that plan, that purpose. In Jesus' name I pray. Amen.

Read Psalm 139:1-18. What does God know about each of us?

_____

_____

_____

_____

How does He know these things (see verses 13-16)?

_____

_____

_____

_____

_____

Where is God? When does He think of us (see verses 7-12,17-18)?

_____

_____

_____

_____

Now read Ecclesiastes 3:1-8. How do these verses relate to God's plan for each of us?

_____

_____

_____

_____

What does David observe in Psalm 31:14-15, and what does this reveal about trusting God?

_____

_____

_____

_____

Turn back to Ecclesiastes 3. What does verse 11 reveal?

_____

_____

_____

_____

Look up Jeremiah 29:11. What does God tell us about His plans for us?

_____

_____

_____

Father, help me to make the most of this time, this season of my life today. My faith and my hope and my trust are in You. Amen.

THE BIG PICTURE

*Lord, open my eyes to see what You are doing—where You are at work—
in my life and the lives of my family and friends. Amen.*

This week, we're talking about being thankful for God's plans for us, even when they're different from our own. Turn to Isaiah 55:8-9 and Romans 11:33-36. What do these verses reveal about God's plans and purposes, as compared to ours?

_____

_____

_____

_____

Now look up Proverbs 16:9 and Proverbs 19:21. What do these verses reveal about who is ultimately in charge of our lives?

_____

_____

_____

Read James 4:13-15. Who must always be a part of our plans? Whose desires come before ours?

_____

_____

_____

_____

There are many, many Scriptures that encourage us to "count the cost," "number our days," "carefully consider" or "examine" our ways. It's not unbiblical to set goals or make plans. But we must always remember that we don't see the big picture; God does. We don't have all the facts; God does. We don't know the beginning from the end; God does. So all of our plans for the future, all of our hopes and dreams, all of our goals need to be inspired by Him, led by Him, submitted to Him, surrendered to Him. According to Romans 12:1-2, how can we align our will with God's will? How can we know what His will is for us?

_____

_____

_____

What are some specific ways that we can we renew our minds?

_____

_____

_____

Look up 1 Thessalonians 5:16-18. What three things do we know—beyond a shadow of a doubt—are God's will for us?

1. _____
2. _____
3. _____

What declarations did the psalmist make in Psalms 40:8 and 119:47?

_____

_____

_____

Lord God, Your ways are so much higher than mine, Your plans and purposes so far beyond what I can comprehend. Be glorified in my life. Amen.

GOD'S ASSURANCE

Day
4

Father, I want to pray as Your Son prayed: Not my will but Yours be done. With all that I am and all that I hope to be, I trust You. Amen.

Look up Proverbs 3:5-6. What three things are we urged to do?

1. _____
2. _____
3. _____

What will God do (see verse 6)?

_____

_____

_____

_____

Read Psalm 37. What promise do we find in verse 4?

_____

_____

_____

_____

When we delight in the Lord, we learn to love Him wholeheartedly and trust Him completely. We learn to love what He loves and desire for ourselves what He desires for us. And we find, as poet Elizabeth Barrett Browning once observed, "God's gifts put man's best dreams to shame." What gift will God give to those who delight in Him (see verses 18,37)?

_____

_____

_____

_____

Why should we not worry or be angry or be envious when we see sinners prosper (see verses 1-2,9-10,20)?

_____

_____

_____

What assurance are we given in verses 23-24?

_____

_____

_____

_____

Why does God help the righteous (see verses 39-40)?

_____

_____

_____

_____

In all the big things and the small things, in the major life events and in the minor interruptions and disruptions that are a part of our daily lives, God is in control. We can thank Him for the work that He is accomplishing in us and through us, even if we can't see it or feel it, even if it doesn't make sense to us or it's not what we would do. He loves us more than we can comprehend. And everything He does is for our good.

Lord Jesus, I delight in You. May You delight in me, too. Draw me into a deeper faith, a deeper trust as I walk in obedience to You. Amen.

GOD'S DESIGN

Day **5**

Father, I trust You. I believe every one of Your promises. You are always true to Your Word. Amen.

This week, we've been talking about the sovereignty of God. Turn to Isaiah 54:16-17. According to these verses, what is God's role in the testing and chastening that we experience?

_____

_____

_____

_____

What does He promise the outcome will be?

_____

_____

_____

_____

In Genesis 37, we read that Joseph was born to a life of wealth and privilege. He was not only his father's favorite son, but he was also handsome and gifted. He knew from an early age that God had a call on his life. But things didn't quite turn out the way Joseph expected. His older brothers bitterly resented him for the place he held in his father's heart. They didn't care for the way the "goody two-shoes" always showed them up. His self-confidence was irritating. One day, they had had enough. They ambushed Joseph and threw him in a pit. They talked about killing him, but ended up selling him into slavery instead. His own brothers!

The son of privilege was taken hundreds of miles from home to become a slave in Egypt. Later, he was accused of a crime he didn't commit and was thrown into prison for three long years (see Genesis 39). Alone, abandoned, forgotten . . . and yet not. For God was with him! God gave Joseph the ability to interpret Pharaoh's prophetic dream, and in one day Joseph went from prisoner to prime minister! Years later, when his brothers came to Egypt to buy food during the famine, they were astonished to find Joseph in command (see Genesis 41–45).

Joseph was able to let go of any hurt and bitterness he might have felt over their betrayal. He saw God's hand in everything that had happened to him. He knew the call on his life had indeed been fulfilled.

Read Genesis 50:20. What did Joseph explain to his family?

_____

_____

_____

One day, we will see that even though things didn't go according to our plans and some of our hopes and dreams went unfulfilled, and even though others have intended to harm us and Satan has attempted to destroy us, God has been working everything together for our good!

Lord, I declare that what others meant for evil, You meant for good. You have been and will always be my Rock, my Refuge, my Strength. Amen.

REFLECTION AND APPLICATION

Day
6

Lord Jesus, You have not led me this far only to leave me now. I know You will continue to walk with me on this journey—every step of the way. Amen.

Earlier, you set some goals—physical, mental, emotional and spiritual. We're now more than halfway through this 12-week study. It's time to check your progress! Review the goals you recorded in Week 2 and then answer the questions below. Which of these statements best reflects where you are in regard to each of your goals?

Physical	Mental	Emotional	Spiritual	
				I'm on the right track. I'm going to make it!
				I can do it, but I'll have to work harder!
				I've met my goal. I need a new one!
				I need to adjust my goal to something more doable for me right now.

Below, rerecord your goals and recommit yourself to accomplishing them. If you need to be flexible and adjust your goals or set some new ones, use this space to record them. (For ideas or suggestions, talk to your group leader.) After each goal, briefly record what you need to do (or do differently) to reach it.

Physical health

_____

_____

_____

_____

Mental health

_____

_____

_____

Emotional health

_____

_____

_____

Spiritual health

_____

_____

_____

Write this week's Scripture verse (and its Scripture reference) from memory in the space provided below.

_____

_____

_____

Lord, accomplish Your plans and purposes for me, in me, and through me. In Jesus' name I pray. Amen.

Day 7 — REFLECTION AND APPLICATION

Holy Spirit, bring to my remembrance all the things that You have taught me this week—all the things for which I have to be thankful. Amen.

Take some time to list the things you are thankful for this week. As you make your list, remember to keep it simple, keep it honest, keep it personal, and keep it specific.

_____

_____

_____

In what ways can you thank God for His sovereignty over the things you have experienced in your past?

_____

_____

_____

_____

In what ways can you thank God that He is sovereign over the things you are experiencing in your life today?

_____

_____

_____

In what ways can you thank God that He is sovereign over your future and has a plan for it?

_____

_____

_____

_____

"To be always in a thankful state of heart before God is not to be considered a high plane of spirituality but rather the normal attitude of one who believes that 'all things work together for good to them that love God, who are called according to his purpose'" (see Romans 8:28) (William Law).

Thank You, thank You, thank You, Lord, for each of these blessings and countless others that You have poured out on me. My heart is full of my love for You and Your love for me. Amen.

Notes
1. Christin Ditchfield, *Praying Ephesians* (Brentwood, TN: Worthy Publishing, 2012), pp. 53-54.
2. John Piper, *Spectacular Sins: And Their Global Purpose in the Glory of Christ* (Wheaton, IL: Crossway Books, 2008).

Group Prayer Requests

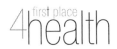

Today's Date: _____

Name	Request

Results

_____

_____

_____

_____

_____

_____

thankful
for His peace

SCRIPTURE MEMORY VERSE
Cast all your anxiety on him because he cares for you.
1 PETER 5:7

A young man once shared that his mother had always been a deeply troubled woman. She was very anxious, worried and depressed. The irony was that for someone who had "trusted in Christ," she seemed to have no trust, no faith, no peace at all. He spent hours trying to reason with her. He tried to show her how irrational her fears were and to convince her to let them go. Over and over he pointed out what the Bible says about worry—that it's a sin, that it only robs us of the joy and peace that could be ours. All to no avail.

Then one day, he saw something that astonished him. His mother met him one morning with a huge smile on her face. All the worry and fear were gone. Amazed, he asked what had happened to her. She began telling him about a dream she had the night before:

> In her dream, she was walking along a highway with a large crowd of people, all of whom seemed very tired and burdened. The people were all carrying little black bundles, and she noticed that more bundles were being dropped along the way by numerous repulsive-looking creatures that seemed quite demonic in nature. As the bundles were dropped, the people stooped to pick them up and carry them.

Like everyone else in her dream, she also carried her needless load, being weighted down with the Devil's bundles. After a while, she looked up and saw a Man whose face was loving and bright as He moved through the crowd, comforting the people. Finally He came to her, and she realized it was her Savior. She looked at Him, telling Him how tired she was, and He smiled sadly and said, "My dear child, these bundles you carry are not from me, and you have no need of them. They are the Devil's burdens, and they are wearing out your life. You need to drop them and simply refuse to touch them with even one of your fingers. Then you will find your path easy, and you will feel as if I carried you on eagles' wings (Exodus 19:4)."

The Savior touched her hand, and peace and joy quickly filled her soul. As she saw herself in her dream casting her burdens to the ground and ready to throw herself at His feet in joyful thanksgiving, she suddenly awoke, finding that all her worries were gone.[1]

From that day on, the young man said, his mother became the most cheerful and happy member of their family.

Day 1 · A NEW RHYTHM

Lord Jesus, I cast all my cares upon You. I lay all of my burdens at Your feet. Thank You for setting me free. Amen.

Fill in the blanks below to complete this week's memory verse.

_____ all your _____ on _____ because he _____ for _____ (1 Peter 5:7).

Turn to Psalm 55:22. What does this verse promise?

_____

_____

_____

The Life Application Study Bible (NIV) notes:

> Carrying your worries, stress, and daily struggles by yourself
> shows that you have not trusted God fully with your life. It takes
> humility, however, to recognize that God cares, to admit your
> need, and to let others in his family help you. Sometimes we
> think that struggles caused by our own sin and foolishness are
> not God's concern. But when we turn to him in repentance, he
> will bear the weight even of those struggles. Letting God have
> your worries is active, not passive. Don't submit to circum-
> stances, but to the Lord, who controls circumstances.[2]

Look at Matthew 11:28-30. What does Jesus invite us to do, and what
will He do when we accept His invitation?

_____

_____

_____

_____

_____

What are some of the things with which people may be burdened?

_____

_____

_____

_____

Jesus wants us to share our burdens with Him. *THE MESSAGE* para-
phrases Matthew 11:28-30 like this:

> Are you tired? Worn out? . . . Come to me. Get away with me and
> you'll recover your life. I'll show you how to take a real rest. Walk
> with me and work with me—watch how I do it. Learn the un-
> forced rhythms of grace. I won't lay anything heavy or ill-fitting

on you. Keep company with me and you'll learn to live freely and lightly.

Jesus doesn't say that we won't have to work, but whatever work we have in this life will be more meaningful when we "yoke" ourselves with and have help from such a powerful partner.

Father God, still my pounding heart, my racing mind, my frantic pace. Help me to remember who You are, who I am and what is truly important. Amen.

<table>
<tr><td>Day
2</td></tr>
</table>

A NEW PATH

Thank You, God, that I don't have to face a single day—I don't have to take a single step—on my own. You are with me always. How that fills my heart with peace! Amen.

In her book *A Thankful Heart*, Carole Lewis asks:

Have you ever had a season when your to-do list seemed as thick as a phone book? In that season it felt like all the responsibilities and pressures of life would simply overwhelm you. I've felt the same way too. Sometimes, the stress in those seasons is our own fault—like when we say yes to too many activities, or when our sins and shortcomings create messy situations for us. At other times, stress can simply stack up through no fault of our own like so many dirty dishes in the sink. In those seasons, I find that giving thanks helps me simply to focus on what I need to do for that one moment. The next moment will come after that, and then after that another moment will come. Step by step, being thankful helps me walk through a full season of life. My task becomes simply to do the next right thing.[3]

Giving thanks helps us clear our minds of the clutter of negative, unhealthy and ultimately unproductive thoughts and feelings. It helps us identify the lies of the enemy and respond with the truth of God's Word. In Psalm 119:105, to what does the psalmist compare God's Word?

_____

_____

_____

_____

Turn to Psalm 18:28-29. For what does the psalmist thank God (see verse 28)? With God's help, what can we do (see verse 29)?

_____

_____

_____

What does Psalm 119:165 tell us?

_____

_____

_____

Read verse 169. What can we gain from God's Word?

_____

_____

_____

Now look at verse 175. What does the psalmist ask God to do?

_____

_____

Take some time right now to clear your heart and mind by giving thanks for everything you can think of in your present circumstances—

particularly your to-do list. Then prayerfully consider the path you are on. What is the "next right thing" for you to do today?

_____

_____

_____

_____

How many items on your list relate to your First Place 4 Health journey? How is the time you are spending in God's Word helping you do the "next right thing"?

_____

_____

_____

_____

Lord, I commit my plans and my path to You. Order my steps. Lead me and guide me. In Your name I pray. Amen.

Day
3

A NEW PERSPECTIVE

Lord, lift my vision. Give me a new perspective, a fresh perspective. Help me to see opportunities to grow in my faith and bring glory to You. Amen.

We lose our peace when we lose our eternal perspective—when we focus on the day-to-day challenges and frustrations we have and the trials and tribulations we face in our lives. We forget that this life is not all there is. This world is not what we're living for. Look up 1 Peter 1:3-9. First and foremost, why should we praise God—for what do we have to be thankful (see verse 3)?

_____

_____

_____

_____

What else have we been given (see verse 4)?

_____

_____

_____

_____

When we have faith, what does God do for us (see verse 5)?

_____

_____

_____

_____

According to verse 6, what is temporary, only "for a little while"? What two purposes do these things serve (see verse 7)

_____

_____

_____

_____

With what does (or should) our faith in Jesus fill us (see verse 8)?

_____

_____

_____

_____

Why? What reason do we have (see verse 9)?

_____

_____

_____

_____

Father, don't let me be distracted by daily battles or life's trials. Keep my eyes fixed on You and the glorious hope to which You have called me. Amen.

Day
4

A NEW FOCUS

Lord, help me to remember that nothing that happens to me catches You off guard. You are always ready to give me the peace and the hope and the strength I need. Amen.

Look up 1 Peter 1:13. What three things do we need in order to walk in obedience to God's Word?

1. _____

2. _____

3. _____

How do these things help us to have thankful hearts?

_____

_____

_____

_____

What warning do we find in Proverbs 4:23?

_____

_____

_____

_____

Turn to Philippians 4:6-8. How can we keep our hearts and minds from being anxious (see verse 6)?

_____

_____

_____

_____

What will happen if we do this (see verse 7)?

_____

_____

_____

_____

_____

With what should we fill our hearts and minds (see verse 8)?

_____

_____

_____

_____

_____

Apply this to your own life today. In addition to taking "captive every thought" (2 Corinthians 10:5), what else can you do to fill your heart and mind with good things? (For instance, think about your choices in music, movies, TV, books and magazines; websites you visit; people you spend time with.)

_____

_____

_____

_____

_____

What promise do you find in Isaiah 26:3?

_____

_____

_____

_____

Lord, help me to focus my heart and mind on You. Remind me to feed my spirit and not just my flesh. Fill me with Your perfect peace. Amen.

A NEW ATTITUDE

Holy Spirit, bring Your light and Your truth to my heart today and every day of my life. Help me to put into practice everything You have revealed to me—all the things You are teaching me. Amen.

Look up Ephesians 4:22-24. List the three action steps we are given in this passage:

1. _____

2. _____

3. _____

Being worried, anxious, frustrated and stressed out—"sweating the small stuff"—is how we used to live when we didn't know we had a glorious and victorious Savior, a loving and faithful God who is working all things together for our good (see Romans 8:28). Turn to Romans 12:2. What part of us needs transformation, and why is that necessary?

_____

_____

_____

Read Colossians 3:15-17. What admonition do we find in verse 15, and what is our role or responsibility in this?

_____

_____

_____

How can we allow the peace of Christ and the Word of Christ to dwell in us richly (see verse 16)? What is the connection between thankfulness and peace?

_____

_____

_____

We ask God to do His part—to change us from the inside out—and we do our part. We actively, purposefully, intentionally fill our hearts and minds with His Word and His praise. We choose to obey. He says, "Trust Me. Give thanks, even for this. Even in this." We reply, "I do trust You, Lord. I will give thanks. I do give thanks. Even for this. Even in this." Read further on in Colossians 3. In verses 23-24, what important reminder does this passage give us—a thought that will help us give thanks as we fulfill our daily tasks and responsibilities?

Look at 1 John 1:5-7. When we have a new attitude, a godly attitude, how should our lives change?

Bible scholar Jim Reimann says:

> If I truly love Jesus, I will pour my total being into His work and someday I will hear Him say, "Well done, good and faithful servant! You have been faithful with a few things; I will put you in charge of many things. Come and share your master's happiness!" (Matt. 25:21). What could be more glorious than that![4]

> *Thank You Jesus, for working in my heart and mind and helping me to become more and more like You. I want to love You and serve You faithfully in everything I say and do. Amen.*

REFLECTION AND APPLICATION

Prince of Peace, rule my heart. Fill me with Your Spirit,
Your truth and Your light. Amen.

In the days after Jesus' death and resurrection, the good news of the gospel spread like wildfire. The Early Church grew at an alarming rate— at least it was alarming to their enemies. The Church began to suffer state-sponsored persecution. Many of Jesus' disciples were imprisoned, tortured and executed for their faith.

At one point, King Herod arrested Simon Peter, planning to bring him to trial after the Passover. Herod had him guarded by a squad of 16 men. Peter was chained between two of the soldiers around the clock. But in spite of Herod's schemes, it wasn't Peter's time to go. God still had work for him to do. The night before the trial, "an angel of the Lord appeared and a light shone in the cell. He struck Peter on the side and woke him up. 'Quick, get up!' he said, and the chains fell off Peter's wrists" (Acts 12:7).

Anything about that scenario strike you as a bit odd—besides the angelic visitation, I mean? Think about it . . . if you were in a prison cell, knowing you would likely be executed in the morning, what would you be doing? Anxiously pacing the floor? Wringing your hands? Crying out to God in fear and desperation? Or sleeping so soundly that some- one would have to hit you to wake you up?

Peter trusted God utterly and completely. He knew his life was in the hands of his heavenly Father and that one way or another, things would turn out all right. In Acts 4, we read how Peter exhibited this trust when he and the disciple John were brought before the Sanhedrin (a religious governing authority in Israel) and commanded to stop preaching the good news of Christ.

Under the threat of death, Peter and John told the council, "Judge for yourselves whether it is right in God's sight to obey you rather than God. For we cannot help speaking about what we have seen and heard" (verses 19-20).

Think about your state of peace today. Do you have the same sort of trust that Peter had? If so, how can you plan to sustain that trust? If not, how do you plan to develop that trust?

_____

_____

_____

_____

How can you be encouraged to trust God in your First Place 4 Health group as you hear others share their stories? How can your story encourage someone else?

_____

_____

_____

_____

Lord Jesus, because of You I have nothing to worry about,
nothing to fear. I trust You with everything that happens to me today
and every other day. And I give thanks. Amen.

REFLECTION AND APPLICATION

Day
7

Holy Spirit, please bring to my remembrance all the things that You have
taught me this week—all the ways You have shown Your love for me, all the
things for which I have to be thankful. Amen.

Take some time to list the things you are thankful for this week. As you make your list, remember to keep it simple, keep it honest, keep it personal, and keep it specific.

_____

_____

_____

_____

In what ways are you thankful to God for the burdens He has taken from you?

_____

_____

_____

_____

_____

_____

In what ways are you thankful to God for the work He is doing in your heart and life?

_____

_____

_____

_____

_____

_____

In what ways are you thankful for God's perfect peace and the ways you are experiencing it this week?

_____

_____

_____

_____

_____

_____

"The unthankful heart . . . discovers no mercies; but . . . the thankful heart . . . will find, in every hour, some heavenly blessings" (Henry Ward Beecher).

Thank You, thank You, thank You, Lord, for each of these blessings and countless others that You have poured out on me. My heart is full of my love for You and Your love for me. Amen.

Notes

1. L. B. Cowman, *Streams in the Desert,* ed. Jim Reimann (Grand Rapids, MI: Zondervan, 1996), December 1.
2. Note on 1 Peter 5:7, *The Life Application Study Bible, NIV* (Carol Stream, IL: Tyndale House Publishers, 2005).
3. Carole Lewis, *A Thankful Heart: How Gratitude Brings Hope and Healing to Our Lives* (Ventura, CA: Regal Books, 2012), p. 58.
4. Charles Spurgeon, *Look unto Me: The Devotions of Charles Spurgeon*, ed. Jim Reimann (Grand Rapids, MI: Zondervan, 2008), p. 331.

Group Prayer Requests

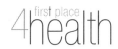

Today's Date: _____

Name	Request

Results

_____

_____

_____

_____

_____

thankful
for His love

SCRIPTURE MEMORY VERSE

Above all, love each other deeply, because love covers over a multitude of sins.
1 PETER 4:8

One of the greatest lies the enemy tells believers is that we can sin without consequence: We can willfully disobey, then we can ask God for forgiveness, and everything will be okay. It's a lie made all the more deadly, because it has a little truth mixed in. God, in His mercy, does forgive our willful and deliberate sins, as well as those we commit unintentionally. But that doesn't always mean there won't be any consequences.

Sometimes the consequences are guilt and shame—a feeling of distance between us and our heavenly Father. Sometimes sin does more permanent damage—to our hearts, our minds, our bodies, our relationships—and we may never be the same this side of heaven. Galatians 6:7 says, "Do not be deceived: God cannot be mocked. A man reaps what he sows."

What better example is there of that verse from Galatians than that of Jacob in the book of Genesis. Jacob's name means "deceiver," and that's exactly what he was. He tricked his brother, Esau, out of his birthright. Jacob showed contempt for his blind and aging father by lying to him and pretending to be Esau in order to get Isaac's blessing. But if Jacob thought he could get away with his sins, he was the one who was deceived. For though God forgave him and prospered him, still, the very sins Jacob was famous for would ruin his happiness later in life. Deceit wreaked havoc on his family life and established a pattern that would continue for generations.

It began when Jacob's uncle tricked him into marrying the wrong woman—after he had slaved seven years for the hand of his sweetheart. Years later, Jacob's own sons would deceive him—just as he had deceived his father—when they sold their younger brother (Jacob's favorite) into slavery but told their father he was dead.

When we look at our own families, we see patterns, too: sinful behaviors learned, taught (intentionally or unintentionally) and passed on from generation to generation; deep-felt needs that went unmet. Even those of us who have relatively "healthy," loving families still have issues to face and problems to deal with on a daily basis. We all have moments when we have to admit that "thankful" does not describe how we feel about our families.

This week we're going to talk about how to break patterns of the past and meet the unmet needs of those we love, even when they are at their most needy, most unlovable. It's what Jesus does for us! (If you don't have many—or any—living family members, you can apply the truths you learn this week to your close friends or church family members.)

Day 1 — DEEDS

Jesus, I lift up my family to You. Be with each one of us every day, I pray.

Practice this week's memory verse by filling in the blanks below.

Above all, _____ each _____ deeply, because _____ _____ over a _____ of _____ (1 Peter 4:8).

What feelings do you have when you think about your family—both the family you grew up in and the family you have now? Take a moment to think about the relatives you have: parents, brothers, sisters, children and grandchildren, grandparents, uncles, aunts, cousins and/or in-laws.

Do you see any patterns—family strengths and weaknesses? Are there specific issues that many members of the family seem to wrestle with? When we identify negative patterns, we can usually trace them back to unmet needs and unhealthy, unproductive (or outright sinful) ways of trying to get those needs met.

One of the ways we can break these patterns is to give to our families the things they need—the things all human beings need: attention, affirmation, appreciation and affection. Although our efforts will be imperfect, God can and will use them to work in the hearts and lives of our family members and draw them to Himself. He is the only One who can truly meet all of our needs. As we give to our families, God gives to us.

Read Isaiah 58:6-12. What does God call us to do for others (see verses 6-7,9-10)?

_____

_____

_____

As we do these things, what does God promise to do (see verses 8-11)?

_____

_____

_____

What will we become (see verses 11-12)?

_____

_____

_____

Read Ephesians 2:8-10. Why should we want to help others (see verse 10)?

_____

_____

_____

_____

Now look at James 2:26. Why is a "body without the spirit" dead?

_____

_____

_____

_____

What do our deeds show?

_____

_____

_____

_____

Lord, use me to bring healing to the hurting members of my family. Heal our hearts, our minds, our bodies, our spirits. Heal our relationships with one another. In Jesus' name, Amen.

Day 2 — ATTENTION

Lord, I thank You for my family. Help me to love them by giving them my undivided attention—the kind of attention You give to me. Amen.

Bishop Desmond Tutu once said, "You don't choose your family. They are God's gift to you, as you are to them." Look up 1 Corinthians 13:4-8. List at least four things in this passage that Paul says about true love.

1. _____

2. _____

3. _____

4. _____

Read through your list again, substituting your own name for the word "love" and thinking about your relationships with the members of your family. How true is each of these statements about you? Put a star next to the statements you feel are mostly true. Circle the numbers of the statements you feel are rarely true for you—expressions of love you need to improve. Make them a matter of prayer this week. Choose two of the statements you circled and for each tell two specific things you can do this week to improve in that area.

1. _____

2. _____

Our families need our love—our time and attention. They need to know that we see them, that we hear them, that we're not too busy, in too much of a hurry, too distracted, or too wrapped up in our own busyness to notice them. Putting down the phone, turning away from the computer, making eye contact, asking thoughtful questions—these are just some of the ways we show our love. According to Romans 12:15, what are two other ways we show we care?

1. _____

2. _____

In order to know what their joys and sorrows are, we have to take time to look, listen, and pay attention. Prayerfully consider some practical, specific ways you can be more intentional about meeting the needs of the people closest to you—particularly with your time and attention. Jot down a few specific steps you can take to meet the needs of your family—and then follow through!

1. _____

2. _____

3. _____

Holy Spirit, remind me to really listen and focus and pay attention to my family. Show me how to make them feel loved and cherished every day. Amen.

AFFIRMATION

*God, You are always reminding me of how much You love me—
telling me how precious I am to You. Help me to follow Your example
with my own family. Amen.*

Mother Theresa once said, "Kind words can be short and easy to speak, but their echoes are truly endless." Look up Ephesians 4:29 and 1 Thessalonians 5:11. What sort of words does God want us to use, and why?

_____

_____

_____

Look at Proverbs 16:21,24. What do words kindly spoken promote?

_____

_____

_____

_____

Now read Proverbs 25:11. To what is "a word aptly spoken" compared? Why is this comparison true?

_____

_____

_____

Read Ephesians 5:19. What is one way we can encourage our families?

_____

_____

_____

In other words, gently, lovingly, thoughtfully point them to Jesus! This does not mean preaching at them or only speaking about "religious" things; it means reminding them that Jesus is for them. He is with them. He loves them. Turn to 1 Samuel 23:16. What did Jonathan do for his best friend, David? How can your First Place 4 Health group help you "find strength in God"?

_____

_____

_____

_____

The people in our lives need to know that we believe in them and see their God-given potential. They need to understand that God will accomplish great things in them and through them. Often, we may see things in them that they themselves cannot see. Our faith in them should motivate them, inspire them, and propel them onward and upward. When they run into obstacles, we can be the voice that says, "Don't give up. You can do it! God will help you, and so will I."[1]

Take some time to think of at least three things you love about an individual member of your family with whom you clash. (If you have more than one relative with whom you clash, make another list in your journal or on a separate sheet of paper.) Read over the list frequently, thanking God for this person who is precious in His sight. You may even print out your list, add photos or artwork and frame it as a gift to give to your family member (of course, you could do this for every family member!).

1. _____
2. _____
3. _____

The more you choose to focus on each person's positive qualities, characteristics and behaviors, the greater your love and appreciation for him or her will be. And the better your relationship will be. And the easier it will be to truly thank God for each one of them!

Lord, I'm grateful for each person You have made part of my family.
Help me to use words that only build them up and encourage them. Amen.

Day
4

APPRECIATION

Father, help me to see the members of my family as You see them. Show me how to love them, encourage them and bless them every day. Amen.

Yesterday we talked about affirming our family members—speaking positive, encouraging things into their lives. Appreciation is a little different. It's thanking them for who they are, for specific things they have said or done, or for the example that they set--letting them know that their efforts have not gone unnoticed. As the writer Margaret Cousins once observed, "Appreciation can make a day, even change a life. Your willingness to put it into words is all that is necessary." What are some ways you can express your appreciation for your family today—in words and deeds?

_____

_____

_____

_____

Those of us who enjoy joking around—teasing our friends and family, engaging in "witty repartee"—need to be careful that we don't overdo it. We don't want to undo the good we intend, by adding a little sarcasm to the end of our compliments. We can steal all the pride and joy, the enthusiasm and the sense of accomplishment right out of someone else's heart. "Wow! You cleaned up the kitchen. Too bad it doesn't look like this every day." "Your teacher says you're so organized and disciplined at school—wish you could be that way at home!" Are we trying to build our family members up or tear them down by such comments? We need to make up our minds. What observation does Proverbs 17:22 make?

_____

_____

_____

_____

We don't want to crush others' spirits. But we have the power to do so. What does Proverbs 12:18 tell us?

_____

_____

_____

Look at Psalm 64:3. To what else are words compared?

_____

_____

Read James 3:3-10. To what does James compare what the tongue can do? Why is this an appropriate image (see verses 5-6)?

_____

_____

_____

Now look at Psalm 141:3. What did David ask God to do, and why?

_____

_____

_____

What imagery in Isaiah 42:3 is used to describe the tenderness and mercy of God?

_____

_____

_____

God sees when we're at our breaking point and offers us His love, His strength, His support. May we do the same for our loved ones!

Lord, remind me of all the reasons I have to be thankful for my family. Make me sensitive to their needs and the ways You can use me to meet them. Amen.

AFFECTION

Lord, You have poured out Your love and affection on me. Help me to share that love and affection with my family. Amen.

Practice this week's verse by writing it (and its Scripture reference) from memory.

_____

_____

_____

_____

Look up Philippians 1:8. What word did Paul use to describe his feelings for his Church family—his brothers and sisters in Christ, and his "children" in the faith?

_____

_____

_____

_____

The most obvious way a person expresses affection is through physical touch—a hug, a squeeze, a kiss on the cheek, a pat on the back, even a high five. Dozens of scientific studies have shown the power of physical touch to promote healing (physical and emotional); reduce stress, illness and disease; and improve a person's attitude, outlook and performance—at work, at school, even on the ball field. Look up Matthew 8:3,15; 9:29; 17:7; 20:34 and Luke 22:51. What do all of these verses have in common?

_____

_____

_____

_____

We know from other Scriptures that Jesus didn't have to touch people to heal them—He didn't even have to be physically present (see for example

Matthew 8:5-13)—but more often than not, He did. Look at Mark 10:16. How did Jesus express how He felt about having children around?

_____

_____

_____

_____

Read Luke 15:20. How did the father express his affection for his returning son?

_____

_____

_____

_____

As we express our affection for different members of our family, we need to consider what is most appropriate for each person and what each one's comfort level is. Here are some ways to show affection to your family today:

- Give your son a pat on the back for a job well done.
- Kiss your mom and dad on the cheek when coming over to their house.
- Ask everybody to hold hands around the dinner table while giving thanks for the food and the time together.
- Sit with your arm around your elderly mom in the nursing home.
- Give your adult brother a warm handshake whenever you meet.
- Give your grandchildren hugs when you leave their house.[2]

Every Friday, the pastor of a local church with a thriving seniors ministry stands at the door to say goodbye to elderly members who have participated in the week's activities. They eagerly line up, willing to wait

10 or 15 minutes for the warm hug or handshake they know is coming. Some have tearfully confided that this is the only physical contact they receive all week. We can't underestimate the significance—the power—of expressing physical affection for the people we love, the people God has put in our family tree.

God, touch my precious family—love them—through me. Amen.

<table>
<tr><td>Day
6</td><td>

REFLECTION AND APPLICATION
</td></tr>
</table>

Lord Jesus, thank You again for my family and all that You are doing in us and through us. Amen.

On Mount Sinai, God gave Moses the Ten Commandments, including this one: "Honor your father and mother, so that you may live long in the land the LORD your God is giving you" (Exodus 20:12). Although it is the fifth commandment, it is the first one most children learn. It is the one they can most readily understand and apply to their young lives. This fifth commandment is also the first one to emphasize the blessings and rewards that come with obedience.

So, what does it mean to honor our parents? Well, when we're children, it may be as simple as obeying them. Whether we like our parents' rules or not, or agree with them or not, or want to or not, we respect the authority God has given them, and we obey. The Bible tells us that learning to trust and obey our parents teaches us to trust and obey God.

But as adults, we are the heads of our own households. We are the "parents"—the authority in the home. We are not obligated to live by our own parents' rules or submit to their authority. We answer (for our choices, attitudes, and behaviors) directly to God. So how now do we apply this passage of Scripture?

When we are adults, honoring our parents means treating them with kindness, compassion and respect. For many of us, it may also mean looking out for their best interests, or caring or providing for them—especially if and when they can no longer care or provide for themselves.

It sounds pretty simple, doesn't it? But truthfully, honoring our parents can be a huge challenge—at any age and at any time—especially if they are less than perfect. (Let's face it, all of them are!) But what if our parents really—and I mean *really*—don't deserve it? What if our parents have been neglectful, willfully absent or indifferent? What if they have mistreated or even abused us?

The answer is found in Luke 6:27-36, where Jesus says, "Love your enemies, do good to those who hate you, bless those who curse you, pray for those who mistreat you. . . . Be merciful, just as your Father is merciful." The harsh reality is that sometimes our enemies are members of our own families, but God calls us to love them anyway. He calls us to forgive them, even if they don't ask us to do so and treat them with courtesy and respect, regardless of whether or not they deserve it. When we do this, we're choosing to imitate our heavenly Father, instead of our earthly parents. And we will receive from God His blessing and reward.[3]

Look at Ephesians 6:1-3 and 1 Timothy 5:8. Consider the relationship you had or have with your parents. How have you honored them? How is your home a "training ground" for your family members?

If your family primarily consists of friends and neighbors, how can your home be a place where they are welcomed and honored? Is there someone in your First Place 4 Health group whom you would like to welcome into your family circle?

Heavenly Father, help me to follow Your example, to love my family unconditionally. In Your name, I pray. Amen.

Day 7

REFLECTION AND APPLICATION

Holy Spirit, please bring to my remembrance all the things that You have taught me this week, all the ways You have shown Your love for me, all the things for which I have to be thankful. Amen.

Take some time to list the things you are thankful for this week. As you make your list, remember to keep it simple, keep it honest, keep it personal, and keep it specific.

Write a prayer thanking God for His power at work in your family—how He is helping you establish a godly heritage and break free from the negative patterns of the past.

Write a prayer thanking God for individual members of your family and what they have meant to you, what they have given to you, and what you have learned from them.

Write a prayer thanking God for the opportunities He has given you this week to bless, encourage and strengthen the members of your family.

_____

_____

_____

_____

_____

_____

"At times our own light goes out and is rekindled by a spark from another person. Each of us has cause to think with deep gratitude of those who have lighted the flame within us" (Albert Schweitzer).

Thank You, thank You, thank You, Lord, for each of these blessings and countless others that You have poured out on me. My heart is full of my love for You and Your love for me. Amen.

Notes

1. Christin Ditchfield, *A Way with Words: What Women Should Know About the Power They Possess* (Wheaton, IL: Crossway Books, 2010), p. 48.
2. Carole Lewis, *A Thankful Heart: How Gratitude Brings Hope and Healing to Our Lives* (Ventura, CA: Regal Books, 2012), p. 71.
3. Christin Ditchfield, *Praying Ephesians* (Brentwood, TN: Worthy Publishing, 2012), pp. 177-179.

Group Prayer Requests

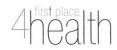

Today's Date: _____

Name	Request

Results

_____

_____

_____

_____

_____

thankful for the pit

Scripture Memory Verse
Surely it was for my benefit that I suffered such anguish. In your love you kept me from the pit of destruction; you have put all my sins behind your back.
Isaiah 38:17

As Christians, one of the biggest mistakes we can make is to run from suffering. Too often we consider our trials and tribulations as evidence that God has abandoned us or that we've somehow fallen from His grace. We desperately want our lives to be happy and pain-free.

As our Creator, God knows that the only way we can be truly happy is for us to become more like His precious and perfect Son, Jesus. Because He loves us so deeply, God is willing to do whatever it takes to accomplish that. He will use whatever He can to mold and shape our characters so that we may be conformed into the image of Christ. And the tool He uses most often is suffering.

Oftentimes it's the heartbreak and disappointment that teach us the most. It's the grief and pain that cause us to cry out to Him. It's the hurt and rejection we experience that give us sensitivity to others. It's the discipline that, while unpleasant at the time, teaches us humility and produces in us the "fruit of righteousness" (Philippians 1:11). God wants us to learn to love Him wholeheartedly, serve Him faithfully and trust Him completely so that every day we become a little more like Jesus and reflect a little more of His glory. As the prophet Isaiah once wrote:

What can I say? He has spoken to me, and he himself has done this. I will walk humbly all my years because of this anguish of my soul. Lord, by such things men live; and my spirit finds life in them too. You restored me to health and let me live. Surely it was for my benefit that I suffered such anguish. In your love you kept me from the pit of destruction. You have put all my sins behind your back (Isaiah 38:15-17).

This week, we'll be talking about thanking God for the "pit" of suffering—especially the kind that comes from our own poor choices—that rock-bottom place we have to hit before we cry out to Him.

Day 1

HE HUMBLES ME

Lord, I don't want to run from the pain or stuff the pain or hide the pain in my life any longer. I want to learn from it! Teach me what You will. Amen.

Fill in the blanks below to complete this week's Scripture memory verse.

_____ it was for _____ _____ that I _____ such _____. In your _____ you _____ me from the _____ of _____; you have _____ all my _____ behind your _____ (Isaiah 38:17).

What often-quoted expression comes from Proverbs 16:18? What does this mean?

_____

_____

_____

_____

What do we learn from James 4:6?

_____

_____

_____

Deuteronomy 8:2-4 describes at least five reasons why God allows times of testing in our lives. What are those reasons?

1. _____
2. _____
3. _____
4. _____
5. _____

Read 1 Samuel 16:7. What does God see that we don't? Because that is true, who is the testing really for?

_____
_____
_____
_____

According to Psalm 51:6, what does God desire?

_____
_____
_____

Why is it so important that we know the truth of our own conditions, our own hearts, before God?

_____
_____
_____
_____

Abraham Lincoln once said, "I have been driven many times to my knees by the overwhelming conviction that I had nowhere else to go." Briefly describe a time during which you were tested. How did you "score" on your test?

_____

_____

_____

_____

Lord, I desperately need Your saving grace in my heart and life. I need Your light, Your truth, Your love. I'm lost without You. Amen.

Day 2 HE REVEALS ME

Jesus, I know You use my trials and tribulations—and even my day-to-day frustrations—to get my attention and turn my eyes back upon You. Help me to look where You want me to look and see what You want me to see. Amen.

Read Psalm 139:23-24. What did the psalmist pray?

_____

_____

_____

_____

What have you learned about your own heart—good and bad—through the challenges you've faced?

_____

_____

_____

_____

What astonishing declaration did the psalmist make in Psalm 119:71?

_____

_____

_____

Read Psalm 103. What should our response to affliction or suffering be (see verses 1-2)?

_____

_____

_____

_____

_____

How can we praise God—why should we praise Him—in the midst of it all (see verses 3-6, 8-9)?

_____

_____

_____

_____

_____

What doesn't God do (see verse 10)? Why doesn't He do this (see verses 8,11,13)?

_____

_____

_____

_____

Why should the truths in this psalm be a comfort?

_____

_____

_____

_____

_____

*Lord, thank You for bringing me to the place where I see my
need to change, my need to grow, my need to draw closer to You.
Thank You for Your mercy and grace. Amen.*

Day 3   HE TEACHES ME

Lord, thank You for loving me too much to leave me the way I am.
Thank You for teaching me to grow in Your grace. Amen.

We've all chuckled over what a parent about to discipline a child has been heard to say to the young person: "This is going to hurt me a lot more than it hurts you." When you're a child, that statement seems ludicrous. But when you become an adult, you begin to understand just how difficult and unpleasant—even painful—it can be to have to inflict discipline on those precious little ones in your care. It's just awful to watch them suffer. How deeply you wish you didn't have to go through with it. If only they would obey!

The Scripture tells us there are times when our heavenly Father has to discipline us, including when He must allow us to suffer the painful consequences of our disobedience, so that we'll have opportunities to learn from our mistakes. Read Hebrews 12:5-11. Why should we be encouraged when we experience God's discipline (see verses 5-8)?

_____

_____

_____

_____

Why does God discipline us (see verse 10)?

_____

_____

_____

_____

What's the difference between discipline and punishment?

_____

_____

_____

_____

What does God's discipline produce in us or do for us (see verse 11)?

_____
_____
_____
_____
_____

Turn to Lamentations 3:22-33. What do these verses reveal about God's heart toward us?

_____
_____
_____
_____
_____

As a loving parent, God is never gleeful about disciplining us. He isn't amused by seeing us grapple with pain and heartbreak. On the contrary, it grieves Him deeply. But He loves us so much that He's willing to allow us to hurt so that we'll learn, so that we'll be motivated to change; so that the next time, we'll obey. Then we won't have to suffer the pain of disobedience at all. What did the psalmist declare in Psalm 94:12?

_____
_____
_____
_____
_____

Look at Revelation 3:19. What reason did Jesus give for disciplining us?

_____
_____
_____
_____
_____

If you find yourself experiencing the painful consequences of disobedience today, don't run from God in your pain—run *to* Him. Confess your sin, receive His forgiveness, and experience His amazing grace!

> *Father, thank You for Your loving discipline and correction. Help me*
> *to receive it and learn from it and grow from it every day. Amen.*

Day 4 — HE TRAINS ME

Lord Jesus, thank You for Your saving grace, Your redeeming love,
Your life-transforming power at work in me. Amen.

Sometimes suffering anguish—finding ourselves in what seems to be bottomless pits—serves yet another purpose. God takes our failures and defeats and turns them into opportunities for us to learn and grow—and train for victory in the future! Look up Psalm 18:33-34 and Psalm 144:1-2. Through all the troubles, all the hardships and all the adversities the psalmist faced, what was God doing?

_____

_____

_____

_____

God calls us to actively participate in the process. What imagery did Paul use in 1 Corinthians 9:24-25, and what was his advice?

_____

_____

_____

_____

According to 2 Peter 1:5-8, what should we be making every effort to do?

_____

_____

_____

What instruction does Hebrews 10:36 give us?

_____

_____

_____

What encouragement do we find in Hebrews 12:1-3? What do we need to do to move on, move forward and make progress?

_____

_____

_____

_____

Your First Place 4 Health group can be a source of encouragement, accountability and support. How can you tap into this resource as you strive to make progress?

_____

_____

_____

_____

Father, never let me forget I don't have to face everything—or anything—on my own. You are always with me and always ready to help me. Amen.

HE DELIVERS ME

Day 5

Lord, I don't want to stay in anguish forever. Come to my rescue! Deliver me, I pray. Amen.

Practice this week's verse by writing it (and its Scripture reference) from memory.

_____

_____

_____

_____

Read Psalm 40:1-3. What will the Lord do for us that He did for David (see verses 2-3)?

_____

_____

_____

_____

_____

How will our experiences—our stories—ultimately be used for God's glory (see verse 3)?

_____

_____

_____

_____

_____

Sometimes it's hard to wait on the Lord. We get impatient. We get frustrated. We get discouraged. We may even despair. Look at Psalm 42:5-6. What did the psalmist tell himself when he was depressed about his particular situation?

_____

_____

_____

_____

_____

Read Psalm 33:16-17. What is it that we cannot rely on to deliver and save us?

_____

_____

_____

_____

_____

Turn to 2 Samuel 22:33. What does God do for us?

_____

_____

_____

_____

Charles Spurgeon said, "Yes, it is true we must endure trials, but it is just as true that the Lord delivers us out of them. It is true we all have our sinful shortcomings, which we all regret, but it is equally as true that we have an all-sufficient Savior who overcomes these shortcomings and delivers us from their power."[1] According to Isaiah 61:1-2 (quoted by Jesus in Luke 4:18-19), what did Jesus come to do?

_____

_____

_____

_____

According to Exodus 15:2, what is God to us?

_____

_____

_____

_____

> _Jesus, You are my Savior, my Deliverer, my strength and my song._
> _I wait eagerly for You. I know You will come to my rescue. Amen._

REFLECTION AND APPLICATION

Day
6

> _Lord, please do in my heart and life whatever it takes to make me_
> _more like Jesus. I want to bring glory and honor to You. Amen._

The Bible tells us in Hebrews 12:6 that "the Lord disciplines those He loves." As His children, we will face times when our faith is tested, our sins are exposed, and our behavior is corrected by our loving heavenly

Father. No discipline seems pleasant at the time. In fact, it's often painful. But there's a purpose in the pain, as reflected in these words by Hannah Hurnard:

> Can love be terrible, my Lord?
> Can gentleness be stern?
> Ah yes!—intense is love's desire
> To purify his loved—'tis fire,
> A holy fire to burn.
> For he must fully perfect thee
> Till in thy likeness all may see
> The beauty of thy Lord.
>
> Can holy love be jealous, Lord?
> Yes jealous as the grave;
> Till every hurtful idol be
> Uptorn and wrested out of thee
> Love will be stern to save;
> Will spare thee not a single pain
> Till thou be freed and pure again
> And perfect as thy Lord.[2]

According to Hurnard, what is the purpose of our pain? What is it meant to accomplish in us and through us?

_____

_____

_____

_____

Why does it have to be so hard?

_____

_____

_____

"Because of the LORD's great love we are not consumed" (Lamentations 3:22). But we will be saved and cleansed—purified by the refiner's fire—if we'll submit ourselves to the loving discipline of our heavenly Father. Briefly describe a time of anguish for you. What did God do for you during that time? How did God refine you? What do you think God was trying to teach you?

_____

_____

_____

_____

_____

_____

_____

Lord, forgive me for the times I've resisted You, rebelled against You and run from You. Thank You for coming after me. Thank You for drawing me back to You. Amen.

REFLECTION AND APPLICATION

Day 7

Holy Spirit, please bring to my remembrance all the things that You have taught me this week, all the ways You have shown Your love for me, all the things for which I have to be thankful. Amen.

Take some time to list the things you are thankful for this week. As you make your list, remember to keep it simple, keep it honest, keep it personal, and keep it specific.

_____

_____

_____

_____

_____

_____

_____

In what ways has God sought to get your attention when you were headed in the wrong direction and turned your heart back to Him?

What lessons has God taught you in the "pit"? How can you be thankful for those circumstances that taught you those lessons?

From what has God already delivered you—or is in the process of delivering you?

How has your First Place 4 Health group been a source of support for you during this time?

"We thank Thee, Lord, for weary days when desert streams were dry, and first we knew what depths of need Thy love could satisfy" (Anonymous).

Thank You, thank You, thank You, Lord, for each of these blessings and countless others that You have poured out on me. My heart is full of my love for You and Your love for me. Amen.

Notes
1. Charles Spurgeon, *Look unto Me: The Devotions of Charles Spurgeon*, ed. Jim Reimann (Grand Rapids, MI: Zondervan, 2008), June 9.
2. Hannah Hurnard, *Mountains of Spices: An Allegory About Human Weaknesses and Strengths Comparing Spices in Song of Solomon to the Fruits of the Spirit* (Carol Stream, IL: Tyndale House Publishers, 1977).

Group Prayer Requests

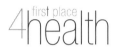

Today's Date: _____

Name	Request

Results

_____

_____

_____

_____

_____

thankful
for His presence

SCRIPTURE MEMORY VERSE
God is our refuge and strength, an ever-present help in trouble.
PSALM 46:1

The elderly woman had lived in constant pain and been bedridden for 18 years with chronic illness. Her husband and caregiver had become ill as well. He needed a wheelchair to get around the house. Day after day, week after week, year after year, the couple wrestled with their ever-increasing physical limitations and all the associated frustrations and complications. If they had grown weary or depressed or discouraged, if they had felt angry or bitter—well, it would have been understandable. No one would have blamed them. But this couple shared such a sweet spirit, such joy and peace and hope in the midst of unrelenting pain and suffering that visitors to their home couldn't help but be challenged and inspired.

One such visitor, Civilla Martin, felt compelled to ask the couple for their secret. How could they be so content, so at peace, when the trials seemed never to end? The elderly woman responded with a reference to Matthew 10:29-31. She said simply, "His eye is on the sparrow." Deeply moved, Civilla Martin went home and penned these words:

Why should I feel discouraged, why should the shadows come,
Why should my heart be lonely, and long for heaven and home,

When Jesus is my portion? My constant friend is He:
His eye is on the sparrow, and I know He watches me.

"Let not your heart be troubled," His tender word I hear,
And resting on His goodness, I lose my doubts and fears;
Though by the path He leadeth, but one step I may see;
His eye is on the sparrow, and I know He watches me.

Whenever I am tempted, whenever clouds arise,
When songs give place to sighing, when hope within me dies,
I draw the closer to Him, from care He sets me free;
His eye is on the sparrow, and I know He watches me.[1]

This week we, too, are thankful for God's constant loving presence—His
ever-present help in times of trouble.

Day 1

HE SEES ME

*Lord, in the midst of my trials and troubles, turn my eyes upon You. I know
Your eyes are upon me. Amen.*

Fill in the blanks below to complete this week's Scripture memory verse.

God is our _____ and _____, an _____ -
_____ help in _____ (Psalm 46:1).

The word "ever-present" means continuous, always existing, ceaseless,
constant, forever. One of the reasons we so desperately need an ever-
present help is because we face so many ever-present problems! In addition to "ever-present," how does Psalm 46:1 describe our help?

_____

_____

_____

_____

What assurance do we find in Psalm 33:18?

_____

_____

_____

_____

Turn to 2 Chronicles 16:9. What does God do for those He sees who trust in Him for support?

_____

_____

_____

_____

Hagar was a woman who had been mistreated by those who were supposed to care for her. One day, she just couldn't take it anymore. Convinced that no one knew what she suffered, that no one saw, that no one cared, she ran out into the desert to die. But in that desert place, she had a life-transforming encounter with God. From then on, she called Him _Lahai Roi_ (pronounced _la-HIGH ro-ee_). Turn to Genesis 16:13. What does this name for God mean?

_____

_____

_____

_____

What does it mean to know God as _Lahai Roi_ in your life today?

_____

_____

_____

_____

Lord, thank You that nothing escapes Your notice. You see my heart. You see the trials and tribulations I face, and You strengthen me. Amen.

Day
2

HE HEARS ME

Lord, I know You see me. You see everything in my heart and on my mind all of the time. Hear me as I cry out to You—as I call upon Your name. Amen.

According to Psalm 145:18-19, where is God, and what does He do?

_____

_____

_____

_____

Look at Psalm 10. What is it that the psalmist fears (see verse 1)?

_____

_____

_____

_____

What does the psalmist learn and acknowledge about God (see verse 17)?

_____

_____

_____

Seventeenth-century monk Brother Lawrence once observed, "You need not cry very loud; He is nearer to us than we think."[2] Look at Micah 7:7. What confidence does the prophet express?

_____

_____

_____

_____

According to 1 John 5:14-15, what confidence do we have?

_____

_____

_____

How does knowing that God is *really* listening make you feel?

_____

_____

_____

_____

Look at Romans 8:26. What happens when we don't know what to pray, when we don't know what to say to God and when we have nothing for Him to hear?

_____

_____

_____

_____

Thank You, Jesus, for listening to my prayer—for hearing the things I don't even know how to say. I do love You. It's in Your name I pray. Amen.

HE ANSWERS ME — Day 3

God, I come before You now eager to share my heart with You— and eager to hear from Your heart. Amen.

Read Psalm 34 in its entirety. What did God do when David called on Him (see verse 4)?

_____

_____

_____

What are some of the things God does in answer to cries for help (see verses 4,6-9,17-20)?

_____

_____

_____

_____

According to verse 5, what do those who rely on God feel?

_____

_____

_____

_____

When our trials seem ever-present—when we're facing a prolonged, continual, constant battle—we might be tempted to feel that God has overlooked us, forgotten us or abandoned us. But over and over the Scriptures tell us that God sees our heartaches. He hears our cries. And He answers us. According to Isaiah 65:24, when will God answer us?

_____

_____

_____

_____

How does Hebrews 4:13 explain this?

_____

_____

_____

_____

It's been said that God answers our prayers in one of three ways: Sometimes He says, "Yes!" Sometimes He says, "Yes, but not yet" or "Wait." And sometimes He says, "No." He asks us to trust that He knows best. What does Psalm 115:11 tell us to do?

_____

_____

_____

_____

God, I thank You for hearing my prayers and answering them. I know that You are working everything out for Your glory and my good. Amen.

HE COVERS ME

*Lord, open my heart to Your truth, Your love, Your peace and
Your presence today and every day. Amen.*

The psalms are full of heartfelt expressions of joy and sadness, hope and longing, courage and faith, that have brought comfort and strength to generations of God's people all over the world. Read Psalm 91. Pay attention to the imagery, the word pictures, that the psalmist uses to describe God's protection. What will God do for us in the spiritual battles we find ourselves in on a daily basis?

_____

_____

_____

In order to receive these benefits, what must we do (see verses 1,9,14)?

_____

_____

_____

_____

What kind of imagery do we find in verse 4? What kind of feeling does it evoke?

_____

_____

_____

_____

Read Psalm 63:1-8. When David was lonely, weary, hurting and/or struggling, where did he go (see verses 1,8)?

_____

_____

_____

_____

On what did David meditate, or reflect (see verses 2,6)?

_____

_____

_____

_____

_____

How did David respond to his thoughts (see verses 3,5,7)?

_____

_____

_____

_____

How can loving God and praising God give comfort, protection and rest?

_____

_____

_____

_____

_____

*God, Your grace is sufficient for me. Your power is made perfect in
my weakness. I trust in You. I want to rest in You every day. Amen.*

Day
5

HE STRENGTHENS ME

*Jesus, You promised You would never leave me or forsake me. You are with
me always. Thank You for the love—Your love—that will not let me go. Amen.*

Living with constant, chronic, ever-present trouble—trials that seem
never to end—can feel pointless. Even purposeless. If we can't see any
light at the end of the tunnel—any hope, any progress, any relief (let
alone victory)—we might be tempted to conclude that the battle can't be
won and isn't worth the fight. But nothing could be further from the

truth. Look up James 1:2-4,12. How should we respond to any kind of trial or tribulation (see verse 2)?

_____

_____

_____

_____

Why should we respond this way? What do trials and tribulations accomplish (see verses 2-4)?

_____

_____

_____

_____

_____

What does God promise us (see verse 12)?

_____

_____

_____

_____

According to 2 Corinthians 4:7-10, what is really taking place when we persevere through suffering?

_____

_____

_____

_____

What encouragement do we find in Psalm 66:10-12?

_____

_____

_____

_____

According to Philippians 2:12-13, on what should we focus?

_____

_____

_____

_____

Author and conference speaker Carol Kent has experienced great suffering, heartbreak and loss. She has had to learn how to live with a "new normal"—a new reality that includes some incredibly painful circumstances that may never change. But as she keeps her eyes on eternity, she finds strength to face each new day. Carol says: "Year after year, God continues to transform my hard places into grace places where I discover surprising gifts of faith, mercy, contentment, praise, blessing, freedom, laughter, and adventure—tailor-made for me with his tender, loving care."[3] This is something God can and will do for you, too!

Lord God, I thank You for all that You are doing in my heart and life.
You are my joy and my peace. You are my strength and my song.
My hope is in You all day long. Amen.

Day 6

REFLECTION AND APPLICATION

Lord, You are my refuge and strength, my ever-present help in times
of trouble. I run to You. Amen.

In Deuteronomy 1:30-31, Moses is recounting the history of the Chosen People and their wilderness wanderings. He says to the people about their time in the desert, "You saw how the LORD your God carried you, as a father carries his son, all the way you went until you reached this place." What a tender picture of God's loving-kindness and constant presence.

The wilderness was a place of testing for God's people—a place where the rough edges could be worn off and their hearts cleansed and purified. They grumbled and complained. They grew weary. Sometimes they doubted God. Sometimes they rebelled against Him. Through it all, He carried them like a father carries his small child. They didn't know where they were going, but God did. He was patient with them. He understood their human weaknesses and frailties. In His big, strong arms, He tenderly lifted them and brought them safely to the other side.

When we feel the heat of the desert—when our souls are scorched by fiery trials and we're overcome by the weakness of our defeats—we can find comfort, joy and peace in the knowledge that we are not alone. We are not abandoned or forsaken. Our Father is with us. He carries us close in His arms. We can also take comfort in the fact that others are walking this road with us. How has your First Place 4 Health group served as a place of refuge for you?

_____

_____

_____

_____

_____

Take several minutes and consider God as your Father—how He created you, loves you, sacrificed His Son for you, has great plans for you, is available at all times of day to talk to you and will always be available to carry you and your burdens. Briefly describe a burdensome time in your life when you felt as if you were being carried in God's arms. How specifically did God help you see your way across the "desert"?

_____

_____

_____

_____

_____

Father, how can I ever thank You enough for Your boundless mercy,
for Your amazing grace, for Your unfailing love? Lord, hold me close
to Your heart today and don't ever let me go. Amen.

Day 7

REFLECTION AND APPLICATION

Holy Spirit, please bring to my remembrance all the things that You have taught me this week, all the ways You have shown Your love for me, all the things for which I have to be thankful. Amen.

Take some time to list the things you are thankful for this week. As you make your list, remember to keep it simple, keep it honest, keep it personal, and keep it specific.

_____

_____

_____

_____

What challenges this week has God brought you through and helped you to face?

_____

_____

_____

_____

How has God encouraged your heart and reminded you of His constant presence?

_____

_____

_____

_____

In what ways can you thank God for the hope of heaven when all of your battles finally come to a victorious end?

_____

_____

_____

_____

"How divinely full of glory and pleasure shall that hour be when all the millions of mankind that have been redeemed by the blood of the Lamb of God shall meet together and stand around Him, with every tongue and every heart full of joy and praise! How astonishing will be the glory and the joy of that day when all the saints shall join together in one common song of gratitude and love, and of everlasting thankfulness to this Redeemer! With that unknown delight, and inexpressible satisfaction, shall all that are saved from the ruins of sin and hell address the Lamb that was slain, and rejoice in His presence" (Isaac Watts).

Thank You, thank You, thank You, Lord, for each of these blessings and countless others that You have poured out on me. My heart is full of my love for You and Your love for me. Amen.

Notes

1. Civilia D. Martin, "His Eye Is on the Sparrow," 1905.
2. Brother Lawrence, *The Practice of the Presence of God* (Alachua, FL: Bridge-Logos, 1999), p. 103.
3. Carol Kent, *Between a Rock and a Grace Place: Divine Surprises in the Tight Spots of Life* (Grand Rapids, MI: Zondervan, 2010), p. 19.

Group Prayer Requests

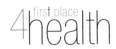

Today's Date: _____

Name	Request

Results

_____

_____

_____

_____

_____

_____

time to
celebrate!

To help shape your brief victory celebration testimony, work through the following questions in your prayer journal:

Day One: List some of the benefits you have gained by allowing the Lord to transform your life through this 12-week First Place 4 Health session. Be sure to list benefits you have received in the physical, mental, emotional and spiritual realms of your being.

Day Two: In what ways have you most significantly changed *mentally*? Have you seen a shift in the ways you think about yourself, food, your relationships or God? How has Scripture memory been a part of these shifts?

Day Three: In what ways have you most significantly changed *emotionally*? Have you begun to identify how your feelings influence your relationship to food and exercise? What are you doing to stay aware of your emotions, both positive and negative?

Day Four: In what ways have you most significantly changed *spiritually*? How has your relationship with God deepened? How has drawing closer to Him made a difference in the other three areas of your life?

Day Five: In what ways have you most significantly changed *physically*? Have you met or exceeded your weight/measurement goals? How has your health improved the past 12 weeks?

Day Six: Was there one person in your First Place 4 Health group who was particularly encouraging to you? How did their kindness make a difference in your First Place 4 Health journey?

Day Seven: Summarize the previous six questions into a one-page testimony, or "faith story," to share at your group's victory celebration.

May our gracious Lord bless and keep you as you continue to keep Him first in all things!

A Thankful Heart
leader discussion guide

For in-depth information, guidance and helpful tips about leading a successful First Place 4 Health group, spend time studying the *First Place 4 Health Leader's Guide*. In it, you will find valuable answers to most of your questions, as well as personal insights from many First Place 4 Health group leaders.

For the group meetings in this session, be sure to read and consider each week's discussion topics several days before the meeting—some questions and activities require supplies and/or planning to complete. Also, if you are leading a large group, plan to break into smaller groups for discussion and then come together as a large group to share your answers and responses. Make sure to appoint a capable leader for each small group so that discussions stay focused and on track (and be sure each group records their answers!).

week one: welcome to *A Thankful Heart*

During this first week, welcome the members to your group, provide a brief overview of the First Place 4 Health program, explain what is expected of the participants at each of the weekly meetings, and collect the Member Surveys. (See the *First Place 4 Health Leader's Guide* for a detailed outline of how to conduct the first week's meeting.)

week two: thankful for each moment

As you begin to work through the *A Thankful Heart* Bible study, be mindful that there may be those in your group who have not done a focused Bible study before. Be sure to take some time at the beginning of this week's lesson time to explain the importance of daily Bible study as an integral part of First Place 4 Health. Give group members who are new to the discipline the opportunity to ask any questions they may have about the process. Recite this week's memory verse together.

On Day 1, participants were asked to describe how and when they first trusted in Christ. Invite volunteers to briefly share their testimonies.

Read the quote from Carole Lewis at the beginning of Day 2. Discuss how having a thankful heart makes us more like Jesus.

Ask volunteers to read aloud Psalm 34:1 and Psalm 71:14-18 (see Day 3). Talk about the physical, mental, emotional and spiritual benefits of a thankful heart.

On Day 4, members considered the relationship between giving thanks and choosing joy. Ask someone to read aloud Colossians 2:6-8. Ask for volunteers to tell how this study can help members live in Christ, strengthened in their faith, "rooted and built up in him." Then ask for members to share some other ways to accomplish this.

Talk about setting goals (see Day 5). On a whiteboard or flip chart, make a list of key words for goal setting. Explain that our goals should be *specific* and *measurable*. Otherwise, how will we know if we've achieved them? Goals should also be *reasonable*. Our expectations regarding weight loss, in particular, can tend to be a little unrealistic. Yes, we'll need to depend on God's grace and His strength to achieve any of our goals, but it shouldn't take a miracle on the scale of the parting of the Red Sea!

With this in mind, invite group members to share one of their specific physical, mental, emotional and spiritual goals for the next 12 weeks, and one concrete step they plan to take toward achieving it.

Discuss the instructions in Day 6 for creating and keeping a Thankfulness Journal. Ask if anyone already keeps a journal or a list like this. Brainstorm different options, from scrapbooks to smartphone apps.

Invite each member to use a journal entry or a spontaneous expression of heartfelt gratitude to finish this sentence: "Today I am thankful for . . ."

Close with a prayer asking God to be glorified in the lives of each one of us as we learn to be thankful for each moment He has given us.

week three: thankful for all things

Welcome everyone and invite members to share any progress they've made and/or any positive steps they've taken toward achieving their goals this past week. Recite this week's memory verse together as a group.

Review the story in the introduction about Corrie and Betsie ten Boom. (If any participants are unfamiliar with the ten Booms' story, you might suggest they read *The Hiding Place* by Corrie ten Boom or view the movie of the same name.) Ask members to think of other stories—from their own lives, from history, from Scripture—in which God took something meant for evil and used it for good. Read aloud the quote from Betsie on Day 1 and talk about the impact we can have in the lives of others, if we will learn to give thanks for all things.

Ask volunteers to read aloud Deuteronomy 31:8 and Deuteronomy 1:30-32 (see Day 2). Ask for volunteers to tell what God being with us, no matter what happens, means? Then discuss how this can help us give thanks, even in difficult circumstances.

On Day 3, we looked at how the traditional wedding vows could be applied to our relationship with Christ—the vows He has made to us, the vows we make to Him. Only death doesn't part us. It's just the beginning! Invite volunteers to tell what we can do to keep our vows—keep our hearts faithful to our heavenly Bridegroom.

Talk about the significance of giving thanks "in the name of . . . Jesus" (see Day 4). Read aloud 2 Thessalonians 1:11-12 and Titus 2:11-14. Ask members to share how they related these verses to their efforts to cultivate a thankful heart—and to their First Place 4 Health journey.

Review the questions about Job from Day 5. Discuss how choosing to give thanks in the midst of suffering serves a greater purpose. Ask for volunteers to tell how this perspective helps us to give thanks?

On Day 6, members read about Paul and Silas and their songs in the night. Ask group members to volunteer which song they would choose as their song right now. Reflect on how God works in each of our lives uniquely and individually—how He meets each one of us right where we are and leads us on from there.

Invite each member to use a journal entry or a spontaneous expression of heartfelt gratitude to finish this sentence: "Today I am thankful for ..."

week four: thankful for His blessings

Welcome everyone and invite members to share any progress they've made and/or any positive steps they've taken toward achieving their goals this past week. Recite this week's memory verse together as a group.

Ask volunteers to take turns reading the verses from Day 1: Psalm 103:12, Jeremiah 31:34, Micah 7:16-19 and Isaiah 1:18. Ask volunteers to share which of these images speaks to them the most? Discuss why it is so important to start our blessing-counting here. Then ask the group members to tell how these verses can encourage us in the midst of the challenges we face in our First Place 4 Health journey.

Talk about the different kinds of healing we need—and we experience—from the hand of God (see Day 2). Invite members to share their own stories of God's faithfulness and how He has healed them (or their friends and family) physically, mentally, emotionally and/or spiritually. Ask volunteers to tell how we can thank God—for what can we thank God—when we are still waiting for His healing touch.

Have someone read aloud Colossians 1:9-13 and the note from *The Life Application Study Bible, NIV* on Day 3. On a whiteboard or flip chart, make two columns: "From This"/"To This." Have members call out answers from the study ("darkness to light") and then add their own.

Ask volunteers to read aloud 1 John 3:1 and Ephesians 3:14-19. Discuss the imagery in the title of the study on Day 4: "He Crowns Me with Love." Invite the group members to list other kinds of crowns (or hats)—good or bad—that we might give to ourselves or we might be given by the world (Champion, Winner, #1 Dad, Diva, Princess, Loser, Failure, Idiot, Dunce). Invite volunteers to tell why the crown God gives us is so special. Discuss how it empowers us to reject the negative "crowns" given to us by ourselves or others.

Ask a volunteer to read aloud Psalm 84:1-2 and 10-12 (see Day 5). Talk about the phrase "no good thing does he withhold." What does that phrase mean? What can we conclude about the things God does seem to be withholding from us (at least so far)? What can we do while we wait?

Invite each member to use a journal entry or a spontaneous expression of heartfelt gratitude to finish this sentence: "Today I am thankful for . . ." Close by reading aloud Psalm 103:1-4.

week five: thankful for our thorns

Welcome everyone and invite members to share any progress they've made and/or any positive steps they've taken toward achieving their goals this past week. Recite this week's memory verse together as a group.

This week's topic is thanking God for our thorns; the difficult people we encounter day-to-day. Before you begin your discussion, caution group members not to accidentally or unintentionally gossip about, judge or criticize people who are not present. Remind them not to give names or identifying details about the person. As group leader, listen for any indications that a member is struggling with the idea of forgiveness (for instance, if he or she has been traumatized by abuse or is now in an abusive relationship). If you suspect such a situation, privately ask the group member to speak with you after the group and recommend the individual get in touch with a pastor, a Christian counselor, a crisis hotline or some other helpful resource. If the individual is in immediate danger of physical harm, offer to go with him or her to contact the proper authorities right away.

Ask volunteers to take turns reading aloud Matthew 22:36-40, Luke 6:27-36, and 1 John 4:20 (see Day 1). Talk about what loving difficult people means—what that love looks like in practical terms, how we live it out in our daily lives. Ask a volunteer to read Colossians 3:12-14 (see Day 2) and briefly discuss the attitude with which God wants us to approach relationships.

Ask for volunteers to share a positive testimony about learning something from having to deal with difficult people—what God has taught them, whether they ever learned to love the difficult person and how that happened (if it did), and what the whole experience was like (see Day 3). Point out to the group that dealing with difficult people can sometimes trigger emotional eating—a coping mechanism some people use when they are angry, hurt or upset. Ask members to share ideas about productive ways to deal with stress.

Ask volunteers to share how they reacted to the statement: "You are a difficult person." Then ask how this affects their perspective on God's call to love and forgive (see Day 4). Point out to the group that forgiving others does not necessarily mean that we should forget the hurt or harm we suffered. God does not expect us to continue to maintain any relationship that is harmful to our wellbeing, especially a relationship that is physically or verbally abusive.

On Day 5, members were asked to consider how they might pray for the difficult people in their lives. Ask volunteers to share how praying for others changed their hearts toward them.

Invite each member to use a journal entry or a spontaneous expression of heartfelt gratitude to finish this sentence: "Today I am thankful for . . ." Close with a prayer that the Holy Spirit will give each one of us the love and patience and wisdom we need to handle the difficult people in our lives and win them (or draw them closer) to Christ.

week six: thankful for His provision

Welcome everyone and invite members to share any progress they've made and/or any positive steps they've taken toward achieving their goals this past week. Recite this week's memory verse together as a group.

Ask a volunteer to share a true story—an example from his or her own life or the life of a friend or family member—that shows how God (often miraculously) meets our needs and provides for us.

On Day 1, members were asked to look up several Scripture passages and reflect on the different ways Jesus met the needs of those He encountered during His earthly ministry. Ask volunteers to tell which story stood out to them—which one challenged or inspired them. Also invite group members to give other examples from Scripture that come to mind.

Ask volunteers to read aloud Matthew 6:19-21 and Matthew 6:25-34 (see Day 2). Point out to the group that we tend to gloss over these familiar passages and think of things like "seeking first the kingdom of God" in broad, general terms. Ask volunteers to tell what "seeking first the kingdom of God" really means—what it looks like in real life.

Have individuals read 2 Peter 1:3 and 2 Corinthians 9:8 (see Day 3). Invite volunteers to explain how these verses relate to our lives and, more specifically, to our First Place 4 Health journey.

On Day 4, members were asked to consider the dangers of wealth and the love of money. Discuss with the group how these dangers can affect people from every financial stratum. Ask volunteers to explain how money can become an idol, even to those who don't have much of it, and why is this so dangerous.

Talk about the blessing of giving, using the Scriptures, questions and answers from Day 5. Share with the group this quote from Christian missionary Amy Carmichael: "You can always give without love, but you can never love without giving." Invite group members to tell why they believe this is true.

Invite each member to use a journal entry or a spontaneous expression of heartfelt gratitude to finish this sentence: "Today I am thankful for . . ." Close with a prayer that God will continue to bless us and provide us with whatever we need physically, mentally, emotionally and spiritually to reach our First Place 4 Health goals and our overall goal to draw closer to Christ.

week seven: thankful for His plan

Welcome everyone and invite members to share any progress they've made and/or any positive steps they've taken toward achieving their goals this past week. Recite this week's memory verse together as a group.

Read aloud Ephesians 1:11-12 from THE MESSAGE (see Day 1). Ask volunteers to tell how this truth affects the way we see our lives, our plans, our hopes and our dreams. Talk about the sovereignty of God. What is the difference between His perfect will (what He desires) and His permissive will (what He allows)? How is God's sovereignty related to trusting Him (see Day 2)?

Have volunteers take turns reading Proverbs 16:9 and Proverbs 19:21 (see Day 3). Discuss the difference between setting our own agendas without regard for God and making plans that we submit to the will of God. Note that one way we can tell if our hearts are in the right place is by looking at how we respond when God interrupts or redirects our plans! Ask volunteers to tell how we can know what God's will is and how we can make plans that honor Him. Ask someone to read Romans 12:1-3, and then invite group members to list specific ways we can renew our minds.

No matter how hard we try to line up our plans with God's, there will be things that we don't expect, can't figure out and won't understand. Review with the group Amy Carmichael's story (see Week 7 introduction) and the story of Joseph from Genesis (see Day 5). Ask what aspects of their stories resonated with the group. Invite volunteers to share stories from their own lives or the lives of people they know that are testimonies of how God's plan for them turned out to be so much greater than their own. Also invite group members to share examples of times God has taken something that was meant for evil and used it for good.

On Day 6, participants were given the opportunity to review their progress toward their goals for this session. Be prepared to help members who are struggling, who need to readjust their goals or who need to set new ones. If they choose to share their struggles with the group, you can encourage a little brainstorming—others can share the types of goals they have set and what has worked for them. Otherwise, offer to speak with struggling members one-on-one, after class. Ask questions and listen to their answers. Try to help them come up with ideas of their own. You can make a few suggestions, but resist the urge to tell them what they "must" or "should" do.

Invite each member to use a journal entry or a spontaneous expression of heartfelt gratitude to finish this sentence: "Today I am thankful for . . ." Close by encouraging members to thank God for what they would normally see as an interruption or disruption of their plans this week.

Direct the group members to be on the lookout for divine intervention, divine appointments, God-incidences (not coincidences) each day!

week eight: thankful for His peace

Welcome everyone and invite members to share any progress they've made and/or any positive steps they've taken toward achieving their goals this past week. Recite this week's memory verse together as a group.

Review with the group the story in the introduction to this week. If you can, bring in a black towel or a piece of fabric tied up like a bundle as a visual reminder. On a whiteboard or flip chart, have members name the bundles (worries or fears) they're most tempted to pick up. Ask a volunteer to tell how we can lay them at Jesus' feet, and invite other group members to tell what we can do if we're having trouble letting go.

Have someone read aloud Matthew 11:28-30 (see Day 1). Ask someone to explain why having Jesus as a partner in life is such a good thing. If you can, share an example of how you were able to "clear out the clutter" (the stress of your to-do list) by giving thanks and seeing clearly "the next right thing" to do (see Day 2). Invite members to share their stories, too.

Invite someone to read aloud 1 Peter 1:3-9 (see Day 3). Ask a volunteer to explain why keeping our eternal perspective is so important in all of this.

On Day 4, participants were asked to read 1 Peter 1:13 and identify three things we need to do to walk in obedience to God's Word. Ask them to share their answers. Then discuss how we can apply these points to our First Place 4 Health journey.

Invite members to share the strategies they came up with to guard their hearts and minds—to put good things in and keep bad things out—and whether the strategies helped them to be more focused and more thankful.

Read aloud Colossians 3:15-17 and Colossians 3:23-24 (see Day 5). Talk about how these verses encourage us to handle our daily stresses and experience God's peace. Ask if anyone tried any of these strategies during the week and how it (or they) helped them to handle stress and experience God's peace.

Invite each member to use a journal entry or a spontaneous expression of heartfelt gratitude to finish this sentence: "Today I am thankful for . . ." Close with a prayer for God's peace to flood the hearts and minds of each person present. As they leave, ask members to bless each other with the words of Jesus: "Peace be with you"; and then to reply with, "And also with you."

week nine: thankful for His love

Welcome everyone and invite members to share any progress they've made and/or any positive steps they've taken toward achieving their goals this past week. Recite this week's memory verse together as a group.

On Day 1, members were asked to think about and identify unhealthy or even sinful patterns of behavior that they can see in their families. Invite volunteers to share their observations in general terms. (They don't necessarily need to share all their family secrets!)

Talk about how relational stress and family drama can derail our best efforts to make healthy choices. (see Day 2). Encourage members to share the tips and strategies they use to deal with these challenges or help prevent them in the future. Point out to the group members that sometimes we do need to set boundaries so that ongoing drama doesn't repeatedly keep us from making healthy choices (making it to the gym, attending our weekly First Place 4 Health meetings, and so on). But with God's help, we can still find ways to express our love and care for the needs of others without derailing ourselves in the process.

Ask the group members which of the four basic needs discussed this week—attention, affirmation, appreciation and affection—they have the hardest time meeting and why (see Days 2-5). Invite volunteers to share how they have tried to meet these needs in their own lives; how they can be more intentional, more purposeful in getting their own needs met biblically; and how they can be more intentional, more purposeful in biblically meeting the needs of others.

Ask someone to read aloud Proverbs 12:18 (see Day 4). Invite members to share examples of how words of truth, words of encouragement, and words of affirmation or appreciation have been healing in their own lives. They may also choose to share how God has given them the right words to speak at the right time to bring healing to others.

Invite each member to use a journal entry or a spontaneous expression of heartfelt gratitude to finish this sentence: "Today I am thankful for . . ." Close by reminding participants that they are not alone! They have you and the other members of the group to call on if they need help or prayer or encouragement. All they have to do is ask.

week ten: thankful for the pit

Welcome everyone and invite members to share any progress they've made and/or any positive steps they've taken toward achieving their goals this past week. Recite this week's memory verse together as a group.

On Day 1, members were asked to consider the significance of times of testing. Ask a volunteer to read aloud Deuteronomy 8:2-4. With the group, review the reasons why God allows times of testing (to humble us, to reveal what is in our hearts, to make us hungry for Him, to feed us with Himself, and to teach us that our lives are in Him.) Ask volunteers to tell how we can relate these verses to our First Place 4 Health journey—to our struggles with obedience and self-discipline when it comes to making healthy choices. Make sure the group members understand that Jesus is our true source of nourishment and strength.

Ask for volunteers to read aloud Psalm 103:1-6 and 8-13 (see Day 2). Discuss their responses to the questions on these verses.

On Day 4, members were encouraged to consider how past failures and defeats (the time we spend in the pit) can help teach us and train us for future battles. Invite volunteers to share examples of what we can learn from times of anguish.

Read aloud Psalm 40:1-3 (see Day 5). Ask group members to explain how we can hold on to this hope when we feel stuck in the pit, how we can keep from giving in to discouragement and despair. Discuss practical things we can do to remind ourselves of God's truth—His promise to come to our rescue.

Ask if reading the poem about the purpose of God's discipline by Hannah Hurnard (see Day 6) changed anyone's perspective on times of testing and troubles.

Invite each member to use a journal entry or a spontaneous expression of heartfelt gratitude to finish this sentence: "Today I am thankful for . . ."

week eleven: thankful for His presence

Welcome everyone and invite members to share any progress they've made and/or any positive steps they've taken toward achieving their goals this past week. Recite this week's memory verse together as a group.

If you have extra time to prepare this week, cut out some simple bird shapes from colored construction paper. Print out and paste on top of each bird shape the phrase from the hymn in this week's introduction: "His eye is on the sparrow, and I know He watches me." Give one to each member to put on the refrigerator or use as a bookmark. (You might also play a recording of the hymn and invite members to sing along.)

Ask volunteers to share some of the challenges that seem "ever-present" in their lives and how they deal with them.

Have a volunteer read aloud Genesis 16:13 (see Day 1). On a whiteboard or flip chart, invite the group members to list the names of God found in the Scriptures (the Good Shepherd, the Helper, the Ancient of Days, the Solid Rock, the Spirit of Truth, my Hiding Place, my Healer, my Provider, Wonderful Counselor, Everlasting Father, Prince of Peace). When the list is finished, ask each member to share the name of God that is most meaningful to him or her today and to tell why that name is most meaningful.

Take turns reading aloud Scriptures from Day 5: James 1:2-4,12; 2 Corinthians 4:7-10; Psalm 66:10-12. Talk about what focusing on what is unseen—what is eternal—in the midst of ever-present trials and tribulations means and how it helps us keep things in perspective.

Ask if anyone would like to describe a problem or crisis in the past that he or she has come through and now has some perspective on. Ask the volunteer to tell what God taught them through that trial and what blessing, or benefit, they can identify. Discuss how reflecting on what God has done for us in the past can help us trust Him in the present.

Invite each member to use a journal entry or a spontaneous expression of heartfelt gratitude to finish this sentence: "Today I am thankful for . . ." Close with a prayer thanking God for His constant presence and asking Him to be with each member during this last week to help them finish this session—this part of their lifelong journey—strong!

week twelve: time to celebrate!

Even though most of your meeting this week will be a victory celebration, take some time at the beginning of the meeting to talk about how much God loves each person in the group and how each of us is called to love our brothers and sisters in Christ. (See "Planning a Victory Celebration" in the *First Place 4 Health Leader's Guide* for ideas about throwing a successful celebration for your group.)

For the rest of the study time, allow each member to tell his or her *A Thankful Heart* story. Give members an equal opportunity to share the goals they set for themselves at the beginning of the session and talk about the challenges and good things God has done for them throughout the process. Don't allow the more talkative group members to monopolize all the time. Even the quiet members need an opportunity to share their stories and successes! Even those who have not met their goals have still been part of the journey, so allow them to share and talk about why they did not succeed.

Making a commitment to continue in First Place 4 Health is an important part of victory. Be sure to talk about your group's future plans, and make each person feel welcome to continue to journey with you.

End your victory celebration by reading aloud this exhortation from Scripture: "Let the message about Christ, in all its richness, fill your lives. Teach and counsel each other with all the wisdom he gives. Sing psalms and hymns and spiritual songs to God with thankful hearts. And whatever you do or say, do it as a representative of the Lord Jesus, giving thanks through him to God the Father" (Colossians 3:16-17, *NLT*).

First Place 4 Health menu plans

Each menu plan is based on approximately 1,400 to 1,500 calories per day. All recipe and menu exchanges were determined using the Master-Cook software, a program that accesses a database containing more than 6,000 food items prepared using the United States Department of Agriculture (USDA) publications and information from food manufacturers. As with any nutritional program, MasterCook calculates the nutritional values of the recipes based on ingredients. Nutrition may vary due to how the food is prepared, where the food comes from, soil content, season, ripeness, processing and method of preparation. For these reasons, please use the recipes and menu plans as approximate guides. Consult a physician and/or a registered dietitian before starting a weight-loss program.

For those who need more calories, add the following to the 1,400-calorie plan:

- 1,800 calories: 2 ounce equivalent of meat, 3 ounce equivalent of bread, ½ cup vegetable serving, 1 tsp. fat

- 2,000 calories: 2 ounce equivalent of meat, 4 ounce equivalent of bread, ½ cup vegetable serving, 3 tsp. fat

- 2,200 calories: 2 ounce equivalent of meat, 5 ounce equivalent of bread, ½ cup vegetable serving, ½ cup fruit serving, 5 tsp. fat

- 2,400 calories: 2 ounce equivalent of meat, 6 ounce equivalent of bread, 1 cup vegetable serving, ½ cup fruit serving, 6 tsp. fat

First Week Grocery List

Produce

- ❑ apples
- ❑ baby spinach leaves
- ❑ berries
- ❑ cabbage with carrots slaw mix
- ❑ cantaloupe
- ❑ carrots
- ❑ celery
- ❑ cilantro
- ❑ cucumbers
- ❑ garlic
- ❑ grapefruit
- ❑ mushrooms
- ❑ onions
- ❑ oregano
- ❑ parsley
- ❑ peach
- ❑ pears
- ❑ red grapes
- ❑ red onions
- ❑ red potatoes
- ❑ red/yellow tomatoes
- ❑ romaine lettuce
- ❑ spring mix salad
- ❑ strawberries
- ❑ zucchini

Baking/Cooking Products

- ❑ cornstarch
- ❑ nonstick cooking spray
- ❑ olive oil, extra-virgin
- ❑ red cooking wine

Spices

- ❑ cumin
- ❑ five-spice powder
- ❑ nutmeg
- ❑ oregano
- ❑ pepper
- ❑ salt

Nuts/Seeds

- ❑ almonds
- ❑ peanuts, dry-roasted

Condiments, Spreads and Sauces

- ❑ balsamic vinegar
- ❑ honey
- ❑ mayonnaise, lowfat
- ❑ Ranch dressing, light
- ❑ salad dressing, reduced-fat
- ❑ soy sauce
- ❑ sweet-and-sour sauce
- ❑ Wish-Bone Citrus Splash® vinaigrette salad dressing

Breads, Cereals and Pasta

- ❑ bagel, whole-grain
- ❑ baguette, whole-wheat or multigrain
- ❑ bran flakes cereal
- ❑ bread, whole-wheat
- ❑ brown rice
- ❑ elbow macaroni, multigrain
- ❑ English muffin
- ❑ flour tortillas, fat-free
- ❑ French bread
- ❑ Grape Nuts® cereal
- ❑ oatmeal, instant
- ❑ raisin toast
- ❑ ramen noodles
- ❑ Ryvita® crackers
- ❑ saltine crackers
- ❑ shredded wheat cereal

Canned/Frozen Foods

- ❑ beef broth, low-sodium
- ❑ black beans
- ❑ broccoli (frozen)
- ❑ cannellini beans
- ❑ chicken broth, low-sodium
- ❑ corn, whole-kernel
- ❑ green beans, cut
- ❑ Lean Cuisine Grilled Chicken Caesar Pasta Bowl®
- ❑ Mandarin oranges
- ❑ oriental stir-fry vegetables
- ❑ pineapple chunks, in juice
- ❑ red bell peppers, roasted
- ❑ spinach
- ❑ tomatoes, diced and no-salt added
- ❑ tomatoes, Italian-style and diced
- ❑ tomato paste

Dairy Products

- ❑ cream cheese, lowfat
- ❑ feta cheese, reduced-fat
- ❑ margarine, light
- ❑ milk, nonfat
- ❑ Monterey Jack cheese with jalapeño peppers
- ❑ mozzarella cheese, reduced-fat
- ❑ Parmesan cheese
- ❑ string cheese
- ❑ yogurt, pineapple-flavored nonfat

Juices

- ❑ lemon juice
- ❑ lime juice
- ❑ tomato juice

Meat and Poultry

- ❑ Alaskan salmon fillets, wild
- ❑ bay scallops
- ❑ chicken breast
- ❑ chicken thighs
- ❑ chuck roast, lean
- ❑ egg whites
- ❑ eggs
- ❑ roast beef, lean sliced
- ❑ turkey bacon

First Week Meals and Recipes

DAY 1

Breakfast

½ cup shredded wheat cereal with 1 cup nonfat milk

1 slice raisin toast with 1 tbsp. lowfat cream cheese and 1 sliced peach

Nutritional Information: 334 calories; 7g fat; 14g protein; 57g carbohydrate; 6g dietary fiber; 20mg cholesterol; 272mg sodium.

Lunch

1 (1-oz.) pkg. dry-roasted peanuts
2 tubes string cheese
8 Ryvita® crackers

4 oz. tomato juice
1 medium apple or pear

Nutritional Information: 469 calories; 20g fat; 25g protein; 50g carbohydrate; 12g dietary fiber; 20mg cholesterol; 998mg sodium.

Dinner

Crustless Spinach Quiche

(1) 10-oz. pkg. frozen chopped spinach, thawed and well drained
1 cup reduced-fat mozzarella cheese, shredded
4 eggs, plus 2 egg whites, lightly beaten (or 1½ cups egg substitute)

1 tbsp. onion, minced
¼ tsp. nutmeg
pepper and salt (to taste)
2 tsp. light margarine
nonstick cooking spray

Preheat oven to 350° F. Combine all ingredients in a medium bowl. Mix well. Transfer mixture to 8″ pie plate sprayed with nonstick cooking spray. Bake 30 minutes or until you can insert a knife into the quiche and it comes out clean. Remove from oven and let stand 5 minutes before slicing into wedges. Serve with 2 (3-inch) slices French bread, 1 cup cooked carrots, tossed salad (with 2 tbsp. reduced-fat salad dressing) and 1 cup cantaloupe cubes. Serves 6.

Nutritional Information: 522 calories; 20g fat; 22g protein; 69g carbohydrate; 13g dietary fiber; 153mg cholesterol; 986mg sodium.

DAY 2

....

Breakfast
Turkey Bacon and Egg Sandwich

2 slices whole wheat bread, toasted   1 strip turkey bacon, cooked crisp
1 egg

Assemble sandwich and serve with 1 apple.

Nutritional Information: 327 calories; 11g fat; 14g protein; 47g carbohydrate; 8g dietary fiber; 224mg cholesterol; 549mg sodium.

....

Lunch
Lean Cuisine Pasta Bowl

1 (12-oz.) Lean Cuisine Grilled   1 cup carrot sticks
   Chicken Caesar Pasta Bowl®   ½ cup light Ranch dressing

Nutritional Information: 392 calories; 11g fat; 15g protein; 62g carbohydrate; 8g dietary fiber; 9mg cholesterol; 1,208mg sodium.

....

Dinner
Scallops Parmesan

1¼ lb. bay scallops   1 clove garlic, chopped
2 tbsp. light margarine   2 tbsp. lemon juice
1 (28-oz.) can diced Italian-style   ¼ cup Parmesan cheese,
   tomatoes, not drained   shredded

Over medium-high heat, melt margarine in a skillet. Sauté garlic and scallops for 3 to 4 minutes; add lemon juice and stir. Set aside and keep warm. In a separate skillet cook tomatoes for 5 to 10 minutes, until slightly reduced. Add scallops to tomatoes and heat throughout. Top with Parmesan cheese. Serves 4.

Nutritional Information: 705 calories; 10g fat; 42g protein; 110g carbohydrate; 10g dietary fiber; 51mg cholesterol; 1,018mg sodium.

DAY 3

....

Breakfast
Bagel with Cream Cheese and Tomato

1 (3-oz.) whole-grain bagel   2 large slices tomato
2 tbsp. lowfat cream cheese   salt and pepper (to taste)

Toast bagel halves and spread with cream cheese. Top each side with a slice of tomato and season with salt and pepper. Serve with 1 cup berries and 1 cup nonfat milk. Serves 1.

Nutritional Information: 302 calories; 7g fat; 13g protein; 52g carbohydrate; 8g dietary fiber; 0mg cholesterol; 7mg sodium.

....

Lunch

Southwestern Steak, Corn, and Black Bean Wraps

1 cup frozen whole-kernel corn, thawed
½ cup fresh cilantro, chopped
2 tbsp. red onion, minced
2 tbsp. fresh lime juice
1 tbsp. extra-virgin olive oil
½ tsp. ground cumin
⅛ tsp. salt

⅛ tsp. black pepper
1 (15-oz.) can black beans, rinsed and drained
2¼ cups roast beef, chopped
6 (8-inch) fat-free flour tortillas
¾ cup (3 oz.) Monterey Jack cheese with jalapeño peppers, shredded

Combine corn, cilantro, red onion, lime juice, olive oil, cumin, salt, pepper and black beans; stir well to coat. Arrange about ⅓ cup roast beef down center of each tortilla. Top each tortilla with about ⅓ cup corn mixture and 2 tablespoons cheese; roll up. Wrap in aluminum foil or wax paper, and chill. Serve with 1 cup Mandarin oranges. Serves 6.

Nutritional Information: 447 calories; 10g fat; 23g protein; 68.8g carbohydrate; 7g dietary fiber; 37mg cholesterol; 818mg sodium.

....

Dinner

Greek-style French Bread Pizza

2 medium red or yellow tomatoes, chopped
1 clove garlic, minced
2 tsp. balsamic vinegar
2 oz. reduced-fat mozzarella cheese, shredded

½ tsp. dried oregano
2 oz. reduced-fat feta cheese, crumbled
1 (8-oz.) whole-wheat or multigrain baguette, halved lengthwise

Preheat oven to 400° F. In a bowl, combine tomatoes, garlic, vinegar and oregano. In a separate bowl, combine mozzarella and feta. Place the bread, cut side up, on a baking sheet. Top each with one-half of the tomato mixture and one-half of the cheese mixture (don't worry if a little falls off). Bake until cheese melts and the bread is crisp (10 to 12 minutes). Transfer to a cutting board and cut each half into 3 pieces. Serve with 2 cups spring mix salad with ½ cup sliced cucumber, ½ cup sliced tomato, and 2 tablespoons light Ranch dressing. Serves 2.

Nutritional Information: 528 calories; 15g fat; 25g protein; 74g carbohydrate; 7g dietary fiber; 41mg cholesterol; 1,206mg sodium.

DAY 4

Breakfast
Honey and Pear Oatmeal with Almonds
1 medium pear, diced
2 tsp. honey

1 packet instant plain oatmeal
1 tbsp. almonds, chopped

Microwave the pear and honey until warm (about 3 minutes). Prepare the oatmeal with hot water and top with pear and honey. Sprinkle with almonds. Serves 1.

Nutritional Information: 492 calories; 10g fat; 15g protein; 90g carbohydrate; 14g dietary fiber; 0mg cholesterol; 820mg sodium.

Lunch
Healthy Minestrone Soup
1 medium onion, chopped
1 tbsp. extra-virgin olive oil
2 (14-oz.) cans low-sodium chicken broth
1½ cups water
1 (15-oz.) can cannellini beans, rinsed and drained
1 medium zucchini, coarsely chopped
1 cup carrots, sliced

3 cloves garlic, minced
¾ cup multigrain elbow macaroni, dried
1 tbsp. fresh oregano or 1 tsp. dried oregano, crushed
8 cups packaged fresh baby spinach leaves
1 (14½ oz.) can no-salt-added diced tomatoes
salt and pepper (to taste)

In 5- to 6-quart Dutch oven (or large pot), cook onion in hot oil over medium heat until tender, stirring occasionally. Add broth, water, beans, zucchini, carrots and garlic. Bring to boiling. Add pasta and dried oregano. Return to boiling; reduce heat. Simmer, covered, for 5 minutes. Simmer, uncovered, for 5 to 7 minutes more or until pasta is tender, stirring occasionally. Stir in tomatoes, spinach and fresh oregano. Remove from heat. Season with salt and black pepper. Sprinkle with additional fresh oregano. Serve with 6 saltine crackers. Serves 6.

Nutritional Information: 398 calories; 5g fat; 12g protein; 43g carbohydrate; 8g dietary fiber; 0mg cholesterol; 554mg sodium.

Dinner

French-dip Roast Beef Sandwich

1 (4-oz.) loaf French bread
1 cup low-sodium beef broth, heated

4 oz. cooked, lean, boneless roast beef, thinly sliced

Cut bread loaf in half horizontally; cut pieces in half vertically to make 4 pieces. Place 2 bread pieces, cut side up, on each of 2 plates. Top each with 1 ounce of roast beef and ¼ cup beef broth. Cover each plate with plastic wrap; microwave for 30 to 45 seconds until hot. Serves 2.

Nutritional Information: 303 calories; 11g fat; 19g protein; 31g carbohydrate; 2g dietary fiber; 33mg cholesterol; 1,013mg sodium.

DAY 5

Breakfast

1 cup nonfat milk
1¼ cups strawberries (or other fruit)

½ cup bran flakes cereal

Nutritional Information: 219 calories; 2g fat; 12g protein; 44g carbohydrate; 8g dietary fiber; 4mg cholesterol; 301mg sodium.

Lunch

1 Chick-fil-A® Chargrilled Chicken Sandwich

1 small carrot-and-raisin side salad
15 red grapes

Nutritional Information: 477 calories; 9g fat; 28g protein; 74g carbohydrate; 10g dietary fiber; 60mg cholesterol; 1,412mg sodium.

Dinner

Alaskan Salmon with Pesto Sauce

4 (6-oz.) wild Alaskan salmon fillets, fresh or frozen

¾ tsp. salt, divided
1 tbsp. tomato paste

⅓ cup bottled roasted red bell peppers, rinsed and drained
1 tsp. extra-virgin olive oil

7 almonds
1 garlic clove
nonstick cooking spray

Heat grill pan over medium-high heat. Sprinkle fish evenly with ½ teaspoon salt. Coat pan with nonstick cooking spray. Arrange fish in pan; cook for 4 minutes on each side or until fish flakes easily when tested with a fork or until desired degree of doneness. While the fish cooks, combine remaining ¼ teaspoon salt, bell peppers and remaining ingredients in a blender or food processor and process until smooth. Serve pesto over fish. Serves 4.

Nutritional Information: 309 calories; 15g fat; 39g protein; 2g carbohydrate; 0.6g dietary fiber; 107mg cholesterol; 506mg sodium.

DAY 6

Breakfast
1 slice whole-wheat bread
½ tbsp. light margarine
3 egg whites, scrambled

½ grapefruit
1 cup nonfat milk

Nutritional Information: 267 calories; 5g fat; 22g protein; 35g carbohydrate; 3g dietary fiber; 4mg cholesterol; 507mg sodium.

Lunch

Quick and Crunchy Chicken Salad
1 (8-oz.) cooked chicken breast, diced
1 (16-oz.) pkg. shredded cabbage
  with carrots slaw mix
¼ cup red onion, sliced
1 (3-oz.) pkg. ramen noodles,
  crumbled

½ cup Wish-Bone Citrus Splash®
  vinaigrette salad dressing
1 (15-oz.) Mandarin orange
  sections, drained
4 cups romaine lettuce, chopped

Combine chicken, slaw mix and red onion in a large bowl. Add crumbled ramen (save the seasoning packet for another use). Pour dressing over the top and toss well to coat. Gently stir in Mandarin orange sections. Spoon equal amounts onto each of four 1-cup servings of chopped lettuce. Serves 4.

Nutritional Information: 516 calories; 22g fat; 26g protein; 55g carbohydrate; 5g dietary fiber; 48mg cholesterol; 620mg sodium.

Dinner

Hearty Vegetable and Beef Stew

¾ lb. boneless, lean chuck roast, trimmed of fat and cut into ½-inch cubes

2 (14¼-oz.) cans low-sodium beef broth

2 tsp. extra-virgin olive oil, divided

1 large onion, sliced

⅓ cup tomato paste

3 garlic cloves, minced

3 cups carrots, cubed

3 cups red potatoes, cubed

2½ cups mushrooms, quartered

½ cup red cooking wine

¼ tsp. pepper

1 (8-oz.) can cut green beans

2 tbsp. water

1 tbsp. cornstarch

chopped fresh parsley (optional)

In a medium saucepan, bring beef broth to boil. Boil 15 minutes or until reduced to 2 cups, and then remove from heat and set aside. In a large Dutch oven, heat 1 teaspoon oil over medium-high heat. Add beef, brown on one side, and remove from pan. Heat remaining oil in pan over medium-high heat, and then add onion, tomato paste and garlic. Cook for 5 minutes, stirring constantly. Return beef to Dutch oven, and then add reduced broth, carrots, potatoes, mushrooms, cooking wine, pepper and green beans. Bring to boil and then cover, reduce heat and simmer 45 minutes or until vegetables are tender. In small bowl, combine water and cornstarch. Stir well to remove lumps, and then add to the stew. Bring to a boil and cook for 1 minute, stirring constantly. Ladle 2 cups of stew into each soup bowl and garnish with parsley, if desired. Serve each with 1 cup salad with 2 tablespoons lowfat dressing. Serves 4.

Nutritional Information: 434 calories; 17g fat; 29g protein; 46g carbohydrate; 8g dietary fiber; 50mg cholesterol; 906mg sodium.

DAY 7

Breakfast

½ medium cantaloupe, topped with
1 cup artificially sweetened pineapple-flavored nonfat yogurt and
¼ cup Grape Nuts® cereal

Nutritional Information: 183 calories; 1g fat; 12g protein; 34g carbohydrate; 3g dietary fiber; 3mg cholesterol; 153mg sodium.

Lunch

Egg Salad Muffin with Broccoli Bisque

1 English muffin, toasted
2 cups frozen, chopped broccoli
½ cup low-sodium chicken broth
½ cup nonfat milk
2 hard-boiled egg whites, chopped

1 hard-boiled egg with yolk, chopped
1 tbsp. celery, finely chopped
2 tsp. lowfat mayonnaise
salt and pepper (to taste)

Combine broccoli, chicken broth and milk in food processor and purée until smooth. Combine eggs, celery, mayonnaise, salt and pepper in a small bowl. Mix well and set aside. Transfer broccoli mixture to saucepan and cook over medium heat until hot. While heating the bisque, scoop the egg mixture onto a toasted English muffin. Serve with 1 small apple. Serves 1.

Nutritional Information: 493 calories; 12g fat; 36g protein; 71g carbohydrate; 15g dietary fiber; 218mg cholesterol; 648mg sodium.

Dinner

Sweet and Sour Chicken with Asian-style Veggies

8 boneless, skinless chicken thighs
  (about 1 lb.)
2 tsp. extra-virgin olive oil
1 tsp. five-spice powder, divided
  (optional)
½ cup prepared sweet-and-sour
  sauce, divided

1 (16-oz.) pkg. frozen oriental
  stir-fry vegetables
1 (8-oz.) can pineapple chunks in
  juice, drained
2 tsp. soy sauce
2 cups brown rice, cooked

Preheat oven to 400° F. Arrange chicken thighs in the bottom of a 3-quart baking dish. Brush thighs with olive oil and sprinkle with ½ teaspoon of the five-spice powder. Bake, uncovered, for 20 minutes. While the chicken is cooking, combine the remaining five-spice powder, ¼ cup sweet-and-sour sauce, vegetables, pineapple and soy sauce in a medium bowl, and toss to coat. Remove from the oven and push the chicken to the sides of the dish. Brush the remaining sweet-and-sour sauce over the chicken and arrange the vegetable mixture in the center of the dish. Bake for 12 to 15 minutes more, stirring vegetables halfway through the cooking process. On each serving plate, arrange 1 thigh and 1 cup vegetables over ½ cup brown rice. Serves 4.

Nutritional Information: 388 calories; 5g fat; 32g protein; 53g carbohydrate; 5g dietary fiber; 66mg cholesterol; 418mg sodium.

Second Week Grocery List

Produce
- ❑ apples
- ❑ avocado
- ❑ bananas
- ❑ basil
- ❑ bay leaf
- ❑ blackberries
- ❑ broccoli
- ❑ carrots
- ❑ celery
- ❑ chives
- ❑ cilantro
- ❑ corn on the cob
- ❑ cucumbers
- ❑ garlic
- ❑ Granny Smith apple
- ❑ green bell peppers
- ❑ green onions
- ❑ lettuce
- ❑ limes
- ❑ mixed salad greens
- ❑ onions
- ❑ parsley, flat-leaf
- ❑ pear
- ❑ radicchio
- ❑ raisins
- ❑ raspberries
- ❑ red grapes, seedless
- ❑ red onions
- ❑ romaine lettuce hearts
- ❑ strawberries
- ❑ tomatoes
- ❑ zucchini

Baking/Cooking Products
- ❑ canola oil
- ❑ flour, all-purpose
- ❑ nonstick cooking spray
- ❑ olive oil, extra-virgin
- ❑ sherry vinegar
- ❑ sugar

Spices
- ❑ black pepper
- ❑ Cajun seasoning
- ❑ chili powder
- ❑ cinnamon
- ❑ cumin
- ❑ oregano
- ❑ red pepper
- ❑ salt

Nuts/Seeds
- ❑ hazelnuts
- ❑ walnuts

Condiments, Spreads and Sauces
- ❑ honey
- ❑ hot pepper sauce
- ❑ ketchup
- ❑ mayonnaise, light
- ❑ margarine
- ❑ peanut butter
- ❑ Ranch dressing, light
- ❑ salad dressing, light
- ❑ salsa, chunky
- ❑ Worcestershire sauce

Breads, Cereals and Pasta
- ❑ bagels
- ❑ bread, whole-wheat
- ❑ breadsticks
- ❑ Grape Nuts® cereal
- ❑ oatmeal
- ❑ oats, steel-cut

- [ ] panko (Japanese breadcrumbs)
- [ ] penne pasta
- [ ] rice, long-grain boil-in-bag
- [ ] rice
- [ ] sandwich rolls
- [ ] spaghetti noodles
- [ ] tortilla chips, baked
- [ ] wheat germ

Canned/Frozen Foods

- [ ] black beans
- [ ] chicken broth, fat-free, lower-sodium
- [ ] jalapeno peppers, pickled
- [ ] okra, sliced
- [ ] peach slices, in light syrup
- [ ] pineapple chunks (or papaya chunks or cling peaches)
- [ ] pumpkin puree, unflavored
- [ ] tomatoes, diced
- [ ] tomatoes, whole and no-salt-added
- [ ] waffles, whole-grain

Dairy Products

- [ ] blue cheese
- [ ] butter, unsalted
- [ ] cheddar cheese, sharp

- [ ] cottage cheese, lowfat
- [ ] cream cheese, 1/3-less-fat
- [ ] cream cheese, fat-free
- [ ] milk, nonfat
- [ ] mozzarella cheese, part-skim
- [ ] Parmigiano-Reggiano cheese
- [ ] provolone cheese, low-sodium
- [ ] yogurt, lowfat vanilla
- [ ] yogurt, plain lowfat

Juices

- [ ] lemon juice
- [ ] lime juice
- [ ] orange juice

Meat and Poultry

- [ ] chicken breasts
- [ ] eggs
- [ ] fish filets
- [ ] ground sirloin
- [ ] ham, lean
- [ ] Italian turkey sausage links
- [ ] sea scallops
- [ ] turkey
- [ ] turkey breast, deli-style

Second Week Meals and Recipes

DAY 1

Breakfast

Whole-grain Waffles with Berries and Yogurt Dressing

2 cups vanilla lowfat yogurt	⅓ cup sugar
2 tbsp. honey	2 tbsp. lemon juice
2 cups fresh raspberries	4 frozen whole-grain waffles, toasted
1 cup small strawberries, quartered	4 tsp. wheat germ, toasted
1 cup fresh blackberries	

Drain yogurt in a fine sieve or colander lined with cheesecloth for 10 minutes and then spoon into a bowl. Add honey and stir to combine. Combine berries, sugar and juice, and let stand for 5 minutes. Place 1 waffle on each of 4 plates and top each serving with 1 cup fruit mixture, about ⅓ cup yogurt mixture, and 1 teaspoon wheat germ. Serve immediately. Serves 4.

Nutritional Information: 354 calories; 5g fat; 9g protein; 71g carbohydrate; 8g dietary fiber; 17mg cholesterol; 338mg sodium.

Lunch

Bagel Sandwich

2 oz. turkey, sliced	light mayonnaise and lettuce and
1 (2-oz.) bagel, spread with 1 tsp.	tomato

Serve with 1 cup carrots with 2 tbsp. light Ranch dressing.

Nutritional Information: 329 calories; 7g fat; 17g protein; 50g carbohydrate; 6g dietary fiber; 32mg cholesterol; 440mg sodium.

Dinner

Southwestern-style Baked Fish with Black Bean Salsa

4 (4-oz.) fish fillets	½ tsp. ground cumin
2 tsp. lime juice	nonstick cooking spray
salt and black pepper	

Salsa

1 (16-oz.) can black beans, drained
1 tbsp. red onion, diced
1 tsp. chili powder

1 cup chunky salsa
1 tbsp. fresh cilantro, chopped

Combine salsa ingredients in small bowl and set aside. Coat a 9″ x 9″ baking pan with nonstick cooking spray. Season fillets, place in a pan, and bake at 400° F for 12 to 15 minutes (10 minutes per inch of thickness). Garnish with salsa. Serve with ⅓ cup rice, one 6-inch ear of corn and 1 cup steamed broccoli with 1 teaspoon melted margarine. Serves 4.

Nutritional Information: 551 calories; 6g fat; 37g protein; 90g carbohydrate; 13g dietary fiber; 49mg cholesterol; 780mg sodium.

DAY 2

Breakfast

1 cup oatmeal with ½ tsp. cinnamon
   and ¼ cup raisins

1 cup nonfat milk

Nutritional Information: 335 calories; 3g fat; 15g protein; 65g carbohydrate; 6g dietary fiber; 4mg cholesterol; 508mg sodium.

Lunch

Chef's Salad

1 oz. turkey, sliced into thin strips
1 oz. lean ham, sliced into thin strips
2 cups mixed salad greens
tomatoes

carrots
cucumbers
2 tbsp. light dressing

Serve with 2 small breadsticks and 1 pear.

Nutritional Information: 283 calories; 7g fat; 14g protein; 44g carbohydrate; 8g dietary fiber; 32mg cholesterol; 521mg sodium.

Dinner

Easy Spaghetti with Sausage

8 oz. hot Italian turkey sausage links
8 oz. spaghetti, uncooked

1 (28-oz.) can no-salt-added whole
   tomatoes, undrained

2 tbsp. extra-virgin olive oil
½ tsp. red pepper, crushed
5 garlic cloves, minced
1 tsp. sugar

½ tsp. salt
¼ cup fresh basil, torn
½ cup (2 oz.) Parmigiano-Reggiano
 cheese, shaved

Preheat broiler. Arrange sausage on a small baking sheet. Broil sausage for 5 minutes on each side or until done. Remove the pan from the oven (do not turn the broiler off) and cut the sausage into ¼-inch-thick slices. Arrange the slices in a single layer on baking sheet. Broil the sausage slices for 2 more minutes or until browned. Cook pasta according to package directions, omitting salt and fat, and drain. Place the tomatoes in a food processor and process until almost smooth. Heat the olive oil in a large nonstick skillet over medium-high heat. Add crushed red pepper and minced garlic and sauté for 1 minute. Stir in tomatoes, sugar and salt and cook 4 minutes or until slightly thick. Add the sausage and cooked pasta to the pan and toss well. Top with fresh basil and Parmigiano-Reggiano cheese. Serve with mixed green salad and light Ranch dressing. Serves 4.

Nutritional Information: 442 calories; 19g fat; 21g protein; 47g carbohydrate; 2g dietary fiber; 54mg cholesterol; 998mg sodium.

DAY 3

Breakfast

1 cup peach slices in light syrup,
 drained
1 cup lowfat cottage cheese

¼ cup Grape Nuts® cereal
 (sprinkled over cottage cheese
 and peaches)

Nutritional Information: 349 calories; trace fat; 34g protein; 58g carbohydrate; 5g dietary fiber; 10mg cholesterol; 806mg sodium.

Lunch

1 Arby's Regular Roast Beef
 Sandwich®
½ cup celery sticks

3 tbsp. light Ranch dressing
1 apple

Nutritional Information: 584 calories; 27g fat; 26g protein; 61g carbohydrate; 9g dietary fiber; 43mg cholesterol; 1,860mg sodium.

Dinner

Cajun Chicken Gumbo

1 (3½-oz.) bag boil-in-bag long-
  grain rice
1 bay leaf
2 bone-in chicken breast halves,
  skinned
¼ tsp. salt
¼ tsp. black pepper
2 cups fat-free, lower-sodium
  chicken broth
2 cups water
3 tbsp. all-purpose flour

2½ tbsp. canola oil
¾ cup onion, chopped
½ cup green bell pepper,
  chopped
½ cup celery, chopped
1 garlic clove, minced
1 cup frozen sliced okra, thawed
½ tsp. Cajun seasoning
¼ tsp. hot pepper sauce
⅓ cup green onions, chopped
nonstick cooking spray

Cook rice and bay leaf according to rice package directions, omitting salt and fat; drain. Discard bay leaf. Heat a saucepan over medium-high heat; coat pan with nonstick cooking spray. Sprinkle chicken with salt and black pepper. Sauté chicken in pan for 5 minutes. Add broth and 2 cups water; bring to a boil. Reduce heat; simmer 20 minutes. Remove chicken; shred. Reserve cooking liquid. Cook flour and oil in a cast-iron skillet 15 minutes over medium heat, stirring constantly. Add onion, bell pepper, ½ cup celery and garlic; cook 4 minutes. Add cooking liquid, chicken, okra, Cajun seasoning and hot sauce. Cook for 3 minutes. Serve over rice; sprinkle with green onions. Serves 4.

Nutritional Information: 297 calories; 9.8g fat; 18.6g protein; 32g carbohydrate; 2.8g dietary fiber; 34mg cholesterol; 469mg sodium.

DAY 4

Breakfast

Banana Citrus Smoothie

1 cup orange juice
1 cup vanilla lowfat yogurt
⅛ tsp. ground cinnamon

dash of salt
1 ripe banana, sliced

Place all ingredients in a blender; process until smooth. Serves 2.

Nutritional Information: 206 calories; 2g fat; 7.2g protein; 42.1g carbohydrate; 1.7g dietary fiber; 6mg cholesterol; 150mg sodium.

Lunch

Turkey Philly

2 tsp. unsalted butter
1 cup onion, thinly sliced
1 cup green bell pepper, thinly sliced
¼ tsp. black pepper
4 (2-oz.) sandwich rolls

¾ lb. deli turkey breast,
  thinly sliced
4 (1-oz.) slices low-sodium
  mozzarella or provolone cheese

Preheat oven to 375° F. Melt butter in a large nonstick skillet over medium-high heat. Add onion and bell pepper; sauté 5 minutes or until tender. Stir in black pepper. Divide onion mixture and turkey evenly among bottom halves of rolls; top each serving with 1 cheese slice. Cover with top halves of rolls. Place sandwiches on a baking sheet. Bake at 375° F for 5 minutes or until cheese melts. Serves 4.

Nutritional Information: 292 calories; 11g fat; 6g saturated fat; 25g protein; 25g carbohydrate; 2g dietary fiber; 70mg cholesterol; 1,027mg sodium.

Dinner

Easy Meat Loaf

½ cup onion, chopped
6 tbsp. ketchup, divided
½ cup panko (Japanese breadcrumbs)
¼ cup fresh flat-leaf parsley, chopped
1 tsp. Worcestershire sauce
¾ tsp. dried oregano

¼ tsp. salt
¼ tsp. black pepper
1 lb. ground sirloin
1 large egg white
nonstick cooking spray

Preheat oven to 350° F. Heat a small skillet over medium heat. Coat pan with nonstick cooking spray. Add onion to pan; cook 6 minutes or until tender, stirring occasionally. Remove from heat; cool slightly. Combine onion, 3 tablespoons ketchup, and remaining ingredients in a bowl, and gently stir just until combined. Place meat mixture on a baking sheet coated with nonstick cooking spray; shape into an 8″ x 4″ loaf. Brush top of loaf with remaining 3 tablespoons ketchup. Bake at 350° F for 35 minutes or until a thermometer registers 160° F. Let stand 10 minutes; cut into 8 slices. Serves 4.

Nutritional Information: 264 calories; 12g fat; 25g protein; 13g carbohydrate; 1g dietary fiber; 74mg cholesterol; 525mg sodium.

DAY 5

Breakfast

Peanut Butter and Banana on Toast

2 tbsp. peanut butter   1 banana
2 slices whole-wheat bread

Spread the peanut butter on the bread. Slice the banana and layer on the peanut butter.

Nutritional Information: 329 calories; 19g fat; 14g protein; 32g carbohydrate; 6g dietary fiber; 0mg cholesterol; 446mg sodium.

Lunch

Waldorf Salad with Steel-cut Oats

1 cup steel-cut oats, rinsed and   2 tbsp. sherry vinegar
  drained   ½ tsp. black pepper
1 cup water   1½ cups Granny Smith apple,
1 tsp. salt, divided   diced
⅔ cup walnuts, coarsely chopped   1½ cups radicchio, torn
1½ tsp. honey   1½ cups seedless red grapes, halved
⅛ tsp. ground red pepper   ½ cup (2 oz.) blue cheese,
3 tbsp. extra-virgin olive oil   crumbled

Combine oats, 1 cup water, and ½ teaspoon salt in a medium saucepan; bring to a boil. Reduce heat and simmer for 7 minutes (do not stir) or until liquid almost evaporates. Remove from heat; fluff with a fork. Place oats in a medium bowl and let stand for 10 minutes. Combine walnuts, honey and red pepper in a small nonstick skillet over medium heat; cook 4 minutes or until nuts are fragrant and honey is slightly caramelized, stirring occasionally. Combine remaining ½ teaspoon salt, olive oil, vinegar and black pepper in a small bowl, stirring with a whisk. Add dressing, apple, radicchio and grapes to oats; toss well. Place 1½ cups oat mixture on each of 4 plates, and top each serving with about 3 tablespoons walnut mixture and 2 tablespoons blue cheese. Serves 4.

Nutritional Information: 410 calories; 27g fat; 9g protein; 38g carbohydrate; 5g dietary fiber; 11mg cholesterol; 683mg sodium.

Dinner

Small Caesar or house salad with light dressing on the side
1 cup steamed vegetables

Split entrée of chicken piccata or chicken marsala 1½ cups pasta with marinara sauce

Order the above items at an Italian restaurant of your choice. Serves 1.

Nutritional Information: 632 calories; 29g fat; 21g protein; 68g carbohydrate; 9g dietary fiber; 30mg cholesterol; 1,663mg sodium.

DAY 6

Breakfast

Breakfast Parfait

¾ cup lowfat cottage cheese or lowfat plain yogurt
2 tsp. wheat germ, toasted

1 cup pineapple chunks (or use papaya chunks or cling peaches)

Place cottage cheese (or yogurt) in a small bowl. Top with fruit and sprinkle with wheat germ. Serves 1.

Nutritional Information: 248 calories; 2g fat; 23g protein; 35g carbohydrate; 3g dietary fiber; 7mg cholesterol; 24mg sodium.

Lunch

Southwestern Cheese Panini

4 oz. sharp cheddar cheese, shredded
1 cup zucchini, shredded
½ cup carrot, shredded
¼ cup red onion, finely chopped
¼ cup prepared salsa, chunky

1 tbsp. pickled jalapeno peppers, chopped (optional)
8 slices whole-wheat bread
2 tsp. canola oil

Set aside four 15-ounce unopened cans and a medium skillet (not nonstick) by the stove. Combine cheddar cheese, zucchini, carrots, onion, salsa and jalapenos (if using) in a medium bowl. Divide among 4 slices of bread and top with the remaining bread. Heat 1 teaspoon canola oil in a large nonstick skillet over medium heat and then place 2 of the panini in the pan. Place the medium skillet on top of the panini, and then weigh it down with the cans. Cook the panini until it is golden brown on one side (about 2 minutes). Reduce the heat to medium-low, flip the panini, replace the top skillet and cans, and cook until the second side is also golden brown (about 1 to 3 minutes more). Repeat with another 1 teaspoon oil and the remaining panini. Serve with baby carrots with light Ranch dressing. Serves 4.

Nutritional Information: 331 calories; 14g fat; 16g protein; 37g carbohydrate; 5g dietary fiber; 30mg cholesterol; 523mg sodium.

Dinner
Beef and Noodle Casserole

8 oz. penne pasta, uncooked
1 lb. ground sirloin
1 tbsp. extra-virgin olive oil
1½ cups onion, chopped
5 garlic cloves, minced
1 tbsp. all-purpose flour
¾ tsp. salt
2 cups nonfat milk

1 (14½-oz.) can diced tomatoes
½ cup (4 oz.) ⅓-less-fat cream cheese
1 (3-oz.) pkg. fat-free cream cheese
¾ cup (3 oz.) part-skim mozzarella cheese, shredded
2 tbsp. fresh flat-leaf parsley, chopped
nonstick cooking spray

Preheat broiler. Cook pasta according to package directions, omitting salt and fat. Drain. Heat a large skillet over medium-high heat. Coat pan with nonstick cooking spray. Add beef to pan; sauté 5 minutes or until browned, stirring to crumble. Remove beef from pan; drain. Wipe pan clean with paper towels. Add oil to pan; swirl to coat. Add onion; sauté 4 minutes, stirring occasionally. Add garlic; sauté 1 minute, stirring constantly. Add beef; sprinkle with salt. Add flour; cook 1 minute, stirring frequently. Stir in milk, tomatoes and cream cheeses, stirring until smooth; bring to a simmer. Cook 2 minutes or until thoroughly heated. Stir in pasta. Spoon pasta mixture into a 13" x 9" broiler-safe baking dish coated with nonstick cooking spray. Sprinkle mozzarella evenly over top. Broil 4 minutes or until golden. Sprinkle with parsley. Serves 6.

Nutritional Information: 431 calories; 16g fat; 28g protein; 42g carbohydrate; 2g dietary fiber; 61mg cholesterol; 679mg sodium.

DAY 7

Breakfast
½ large bagel
1 tbsp. fat-free cream cheese

1 cup mixed fruit

Nutritional Information: 400 calories; 4g fat; 10g protein; 85g carbohydrate; 6g dietary fiber; 8mg cholesterol; 325mg sodium.

Lunch

Black Bean Salad

2 cups romaine lettuce hearts, chopped
1 avocado, chopped
1 medium tomato, chopped
½ cup canned black beans, rinsed
2 tbsp. green onion, diced

1 tbsp. fresh cilantro, diced
1 tbsp. extra-virgin olive oil
2 tsp. lime juice
¼ tsp. lime zest
¼ tsp. salt
½ tsp. black pepper

In a large bowl, toss together lettuce, avocado, tomato, beans, green onion and cilantro. In a small bowl, mix olive oil, lime juice, lime zest, salt and pepper. Pour dressing over the salad and toss well to coat. Serve with baked tortilla chips and fruit salad. Serves 2.

Nutritional Information: 247 calories; 17g fat; 6g protein; 20g carbohydrate; 9g dietary fiber; 0mg cholesterol; 311 mg sodium.

Dinner

Seared Scallops with Pumpkin Soup

12 oz. fresh sea scallops
1 can (15-oz.) unflavored pumpkin puree
2 tbsp. hazelnuts, roughly chopped
8 to 10 chives, chopped
1 tbsp. honey

1 cup fat-free, lower-sodium chicken broth
1 tbsp. unsalted butter
½ tbsp. extra-virgin olive oil
salt and black pepper (to taste)

Toast chopped hazelnuts in the oven (10 minutes at 400° F) or on the stove in a stainless steel sauté pan (5 to 7 minutes over medium heat, shaking often so they don't burn). Set the hazelnuts aside. Combine pumpkin, honey, butter and broth in a medium saucepan and heat the mixture on low until it is warmed through. Season the mixture with salt and pepper to taste, and keep it warm. Next, preheat a cast-iron skillet or sauté pan over medium-high heat. Pat scallops dry with a paper towel and season them with salt and pepper to taste. Add oil to the pan, and then add the scallops. Cook for 2 to 3 minutes on each side until they are firm, browned and caramelized. Pour the soup into wide-rimmed serving bowls. Add scallops and hazelnuts, and garnish with chopped chives. Serves 2.

Nutritional Information: 430 calories; 17g fat; 35g carbohydrate; 7g dietary fiber; 215mg cholesterol; 460mg sodium.

SNACKS & DESSERTS

(Note: You will need to add the items for the recipes to the grocery list.)

Apple Wedges in Chocolate and Granola

2 oz. semisweet chocolate, finely chopped
⅓ cup lowfat granola, without raisins

1 large Braeburn apple, cut into 16 wedges

Place chocolate in a medium microwave-safe bowl. Microwave on high for 1 minute, stirring every 15 seconds, or until chocolate melts. Place granola in a shallow dish. Dip apple wedges, skin side up, in chocolate; allow excess chocolate to drip back into bowl. Dredge wedges in granola. Place wedges, chocolate side up, on a large plate. Refrigerate 5 minutes or until set. Serves 4.

Nutritional Information: 132 calories; 5g fat; 2g protein; 24g carbohydrate; 3g dietary fiber; 0mg cholesterol; 22mg sodium.

Salsa Potato

baked potato, small
½ cup salsa, chunky

2 tbsp. nonfat sour cream

Spoon the salsa and sour cream over the baked potato. Serves 1.

Nutritional Information: 95 calories; 0g fat; 3g protein; 16g carbohydrate; 0g dietary fiber; 9mg cholesterol; 141mg sodium.

Pumpkin Pie with Toasted Coconut

¼ cup brown sugar, packed
1½ tbsp. fresh ginger, grated and peeled
½ tsp. ground cinnamon
¼ tsp. salt
⅛ tsp. ground allspice
2 large eggs

1 (15-oz.) can unflavored pumpkin
1 (14-oz.) can fat-free sweetened condensed milk
½ (14-oz.) package refrigerated pie dough (such as Pillsbury®)
½ cup sweetened coconut, toasted, flaked

Preheat oven to 375° F. Combine brown sugar, ginger, cinnamon, salt, allspice, eggs, pumpkin and milk in a large bowl, stirring with a whisk until smooth. Roll dough into an 11-inch circle; fit into a 9″ pie plate. Fold edges under and flute. Pour pumpkin mixture into prepared crust. Place pie plate on a baking sheet. Place baking sheet on lowest oven rack. Bake at 375° F for 40 minutes or until a knife inserted into the center comes out clean. Remove from baking sheet; cool 1 hour on a wire rack. Refrigerate 2 hours or until chilled. Sprinkle coconut over pie. Serves 12.

Nutritional Information: 224 calories; 7g fat; 5g protein; 38g carbohydrate; 2g dietary fiber; 41mg cholesterol; 200mg sodium.

Hot Artichoke Cheese Dip

2 garlic cloves
1 green onion, cut into pieces
1/3 cup (1½ oz.) grated Parmigiano-Reggiano cheese, divided
1/3 cup reduced-fat mayonnaise
¼ cup (2 oz.) ⅓-less-fat cream cheese
1 tbsp. fresh lemon juice
¼ tsp. red pepper, crushed
12 oz. frozen artichoke hearts, thawed and drained
24 (½-oz.) slices baguette, toasted
nonstick cooking spray

Preheat oven to 400° F. Place garlic and onion in a food processor and process until finely chopped. Add ¼ cup Parmigiano-Reggiano cheese, mayonnaise, cream cheese, lemon juice and red pepper and process until almost smooth. Pulse artichoke hearts in a blender until coarsely chopped. Spoon the mixture into a 3-cup gratin dish coated with nonstick cooking spray and sprinkle evenly with remaining Parmigiano-Reggiano cheese. Bake at 400° F for 15 minutes or until thoroughly heated and bubbly. Serve hot with baguette. Serves 12.

Nutritional Information: 126 calories; 4g fat; 5g protein; 21g carbohydrate; 2g dietary fiber; 7mg cholesterol; 334mg sodium.

Tortilla Roll-ups

6 (6-inch) low-fat flour tortillas
8 oz. fat-free cream cheese, softened
¼ cup chunky salsa

Mix cream cheese and salsa in small bowl; stir well to combine. Cover one side of each tortilla with an equal amount of cream-cheese blend; roll tortillas and place on serving platter. Cover with plastic wrap and refrigerate at least 1 hour. Slice into 1-inch pieces just prior to serving. Serves 6.

Nutritional Information: 169 calories; 2g fat; 6g protein; 29g carbohydrate; 3g dietary fiber; 3mg cholesterol; 583mg sodium.

Double Oat Granola

2½ cups regular rolled oats
1 cup toasted oat bran cereal
½ cup toasted wheat germ
⅓ cup pecans, coarsely chopped
½ cup unsweetened applesauce
2 tbsp. honey

1 tbsp. cooking oil
¼ tsp. ground cinnamon
⅓ cup snipped dried cranberries,
  snipped dried tart cherries,
  and/or dried blueberries
nonstick cooking spray

Preheat oven to 325° F. Lightly coat a 15″ x 10″ x 1″ baking pan with non-stick cooking spray and set aside. In a large bowl, stir together rolled oats, oat bran cereal, wheat germ and pecans. In a separate small bowl, stir together applesauce, honey, cooking oil and cinnamon. Pour applesauce mixture over the cereal mixture and stir using a wooden spoon until the applesauce is evenly distributed. Spread the granola mixture evenly onto the prepared pan and bake about 40 minutes or until golden brown, stirring every 10 minutes. Stir in dried fruit and spread on foil to cool. Store in an airtight container for up to 2 weeks. Makes 5 cups (10 ½-cup servings).

Nutritional Information per ½ cup serving: 177 calories; 6g fat; 7g protein; 28g carbohydrate; 5g dietary fiber; 0mg cholesterol; 2mg sodium.

Lemonade

3 cups cold water
1 cup lemon juice

¾ cup sugar substitute
lemon slices

In a 1½-quart pitcher, stir together water, lemon juice and sugar substitute. If desired, chill in the refrigerator. Serve with ice cubes and garnish with lemon slices. Serves 4.

Nutritional Information: 15 calories; 0g fat; trace protein; 5g carbohydrate; trace dietary fiber; 0mg cholesterol; 1mg sodium.

Member Survey

Please answer the following questions to help your leader plan your First Place 4 Health meetings so that your needs might be met in this session. Give this form to your leader at the first group meeting.

Name _____ Birth date _____

Please list those who live in your household.

Name	Relationship	Age

What church do you attend? _____

Are you interested in receiving more information about our church?

       Yes   No

Occupation _____

What talent or area of expertise would you be willing to share with our class?

_____

Why did you join First Place 4 Health?

_____

With notice, would you be willing to lead a Bible study discussion one week?

       Yes   No

Are you comfortable praying out loud? _____

If the assistant leader were absent, would you be willing to assist in weighing in members and possibly evaluating the Live It Trackers?

       Yes   No

Any other comments:

_____

_____

Personal Weight and Measurement Record

Week	Weight	+ or -	Goal this Session	Pounds to goal
1				
2				
3				
4				
5				
6				
7				
8				
9				
10				
11				
12				

Beginning Measurements

Waist _____ Hips _____ Thighs _____ Chest _____

Ending Measurements

Waist _____ Hips _____ Thighs _____ Chest _____

Martha - ○ Montana

Katnye ○

Ron Shelby ○○ ; herniated disc
(Sharon)

John White ○

Charlie ○ & Marie

Dee ○ Praise. Cindy

Danny ○

David ○

Mary Jane ○

○ Terry). (+ wife)

First Place 4 Health
Prayer Partner

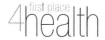

A THANKFUL
HEART
Week
2

SCRIPTURE VERSE TO MEMORIZE FOR WEEK THREE:

[Give] thanks to God the Father for everything, in the name of our Lord Jesus Christ.

EPHESIANS 5:20

Date: _____

Name: _____

Home Phone: (_____) _____

Work Phone: (_____) _____

Email: _____

Personal Prayer Concerns:

_____

_____

_____

_____

_____

_____

_____

This form is for prayer requests that are personal to you and your journey in First Place 4 Health. Please complete this form and have it ready to turn in when you arrive at your group meeting.

First Place 4 Health
Prayer Partner

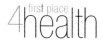

A THANKFUL
HEART
Week
3

SCRIPTURE VERSE TO MEMORIZE FOR WEEK FOUR:

Praise the LORD, O my soul, and forget not all his benefits.

PSALM 103:2

Date: _____

Name: _____

Home Phone: (_____) _____

Work Phone: (_____) _____

Email: _____

Personal Prayer Concerns:

_____

_____

_____

_____

_____

_____

_____

This form is for prayer requests that are personal to you and your journey in First Place 4 Health. Please complete this form and have it ready to turn in when you arrive at your group meeting.

First Place 4 Health
Prayer Partner

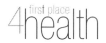

A THANKFUL
HEART
Week
4

SCRIPTURE VERSE TO MEMORIZE FOR WEEK FIVE:

*For Christ's sake, I delight in weaknesses, in insults, in hardships, in persecutions,
in difficulties. For when I am weak, then I am strong.*

2 CORINTHIANS 12:10

Date: _____

Name: _____

Home Phone: (_____) _____

Work Phone: (_____) _____

Email: _____

Personal Prayer Concerns:

_____

_____

_____

_____

_____

_____

_____

This form is for prayer requests that are personal to you and your journey in First Place 4 Health. Please complete this form and have it ready to turn in when you arrive at your group meeting.

First Place 4 Health
Prayer Partner

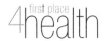

A THANKFUL
HEART
Week
5

SCRIPTURE VERSE TO MEMORIZE FOR WEEK SIX:

[Do not] put [your] hope in wealth, which is so uncertain, but . . . put [your] hope in God, who richly provides us with everything for our enjoyment.

1 TIMOTHY 6:17

Date: _____

Name: _____

Home Phone: (_____) _____

Work Phone: (_____) _____

Email: _____

Personal Prayer Concerns:

_____

_____

_____

_____

_____

_____

_____

This form is for prayer requests that are personal to you and your journey in First Place 4 Health. Please complete this form and have it ready to turn in when you arrive at your group meeting.

First Place 4 Health
Prayer Partner

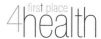

SCRIPTURE VERSE TO MEMORIZE FOR WEEK SEVEN:

Show me your ways, O LORD, teach me your paths; guide me in your truth and teach me, for you are God my Savior, and my hope is in you all day long.

PSALM 25:4-5

Date: _____

Name: _____

Home Phone: (_____) _____

Work Phone: (_____) _____

Email: _____

Personal Prayer Concerns:

_____

_____

_____

_____

_____

_____

_____

This form is for prayer requests that are personal to you and your journey in First Place 4 Health. Please complete this form and have it ready to turn in when you arrive at your group meeting.

First Place 4 Health
Prayer Partner

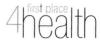

A THANKFUL
HEART
Week
7

SCRIPTURE VERSE TO MEMORIZE FOR WEEK EIGHT:

Cast all your anxiety on him because he cares for you.

1 PETER 5:7

Date: _____

Name: _____

Home Phone: (_____) _____

Work Phone: (_____) _____

Email: _____

Personal Prayer Concerns:

_____

_____

_____

_____

_____

_____

_____

This form is for prayer requests that are personal to you and your journey in First Place 4 Health. Please complete this form and have it ready to turn in when you arrive at your group meeting.

First Place 4 Health
Prayer Partner

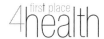

A THANKFUL
HEART
Week
8

Date: _____

Name: _____

Home Phone: (_____) _____

Work Phone: (_____) _____

Email: _____

Personal Prayer Concerns:

_____

_____

_____

_____

_____

_____

_____

This form is for prayer requests that are personal to you and your journey in First Place 4 Health. Please complete this form and have it ready to turn in when you arrive at your group meeting.

First Place 4 Health
Prayer Partner

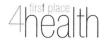

SCRIPTURE VERSE TO MEMORIZE FOR WEEK TEN:

Surely it was for my benefit that I suffered such anguish. In your love you kept me from the pit of destruction; you have put all my sins behind your back.

ISAIAH 38:17

Date: _____

Name: _____

Home Phone: (_____) _____

Work Phone: (_____) _____

Email: _____

Personal Prayer Concerns:

_____

_____

_____

_____

_____

_____

_____

This form is for prayer requests that are personal to you and your journey in First Place 4 Health. Please complete this form and have it ready to turn in when you arrive at your group meeting.

First Place 4 Health
Prayer Partner

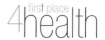

A THANKFUL
HEART
Week
10

SCRIPTURE VERSE TO MEMORIZE FOR WEEK ELEVEN:

God is our refuge and strength, an ever-present help in trouble.

PSALM 46:1

Date: _____

Name: _____

Home Phone: (_____) _____

Work Phone: (_____) _____

Email: _____

Personal Prayer Concerns:

_____

_____

_____

_____

_____

_____

_____

This form is for prayer requests that are personal to you and your journey in First Place 4 Health. Please complete this form and have it ready to turn in when you arrive at your group meeting.

First Place 4 Health
Prayer Partner

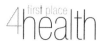

A THANKFUL
HEART
Week
11

Date: _____

Name: _____

Home Phone: (_____) _____

Work Phone: (_____) _____

Email: _____

Personal Prayer Concerns:

_____

_____

_____

_____

_____

_____

_____

This form is for prayer requests that are personal to you and your journey in First Place 4 Health. Please complete this form and have it ready to turn in when you arrive at your group meeting.

Live It Tracker

Name: _____ Date: _____ Week #: _____

Loss/gain _____ lbs.   Calorie Range: _____   My food goal for the week: _____

Activity Level: None, < 30 min/day, 30-60 min/day, 60+ min/day   My activity goal for the week: _____

My spiritual goal for the week: _____

Group	Daily Calories							
	1300-1400	1500-1600	1700-1800	1900-2000	2100-2200	2300-2400	2500-2600	2700-2800
Fruits	1.5-2 c.	1.5-2 c.	1.5-2 c.	2-2.5 c.	2-2.5 c.	2.5-3.5 c.	3.5-4.5 c.	3.5-4.5 c.
Vegetables	1.5-2 c.	2-2.5 c.	2.5-3 c.	2.5-3 c.	3-3.5 c.	3.5-4.5 c.	4.5-5 c.	4.5-5 c.
Grains	5 oz-eq.	5-6 oz-eq.	6-7 oz-eq.	6-7 oz-eq.	7-8 oz-eq.	8-9 oz-eq.	9-10 oz-eq.	10-11 oz-eq.
Meat & Beans	4 oz-eq.	5 oz-eq.	5-5.5 oz-eq.	5.5-6.5 oz-eq.	6.5-7 oz-eq.	7-7.5 oz-eq.	7-7.5 oz-eq.	7.5-8 oz-eq.
Milk	2-3 c.	3 c.	3 c.	3 c.	3 c.	3 c.	3 c.	3 c.
Healthy Oils	4 tsp.	5 tsp.	5 tsp.	6 tsp.	6 tsp.	7 tsp.	8 tsp.	8 tsp.

Day/Date:

Breakfast: _____
Lunch: _____
Dinner: _____
Snacks: _____

GROUP	FRUITS	VEGETABLES	GRAINS	MEAT & BEANS	MILK	OILS
Goal Amount						
Estimate Your Total						
Total Calories						

Physical Activity: _____   Spiritual Activity: _____
Steps/Miles/Minutes: _____   My Emotions Today: ❑ Happy ❑ Sad ❑ Stressed

Day/Date:

Breakfast: _____
Lunch: _____
Dinner: _____
Snacks: _____

GROUP	FRUITS	VEGETABLES	GRAINS	MEAT & BEANS	MILK	OILS
Goal Amount						
Estimate Your Total						
Total Calories						

Physical Activity: _____   Spiritual Activity: _____
Steps/Miles/Minutes: _____   My Emotions Today: ❑ Happy ❑ Sad ❑ Stressed

Day/Date:

Breakfast: _____
Lunch: _____
Dinner: _____
Snacks: _____

GROUP	FRUITS	VEGETABLES	GRAINS	MEAT & BEANS	MILK	OILS
Goal Amount						
Estimate Your Total						
Total Calories						

Physical Activity: _____   Spiritual Activity: _____
Steps/Miles/Minutes: _____   My Emotions Today: ❑ Happy ❑ Sad ❑ Stressed

Day/Date:

Breakfast: _____
Lunch: _____
Dinner: _____
Snacks: _____

GROUP	FRUITS	VEGETABLES	GRAINS	MEAT & BEANS	MILK	OILS
Goal Amount						
Estimate Your Total						
Total Calories						

Physical Activity: _____ Spiritual Activity: _____
Steps/Miles/Minutes: _____ My Emotions Today: ❑ Happy ❑ Sad ❑ Stressed

---

Day/Date:

Breakfast: _____
Lunch: _____
Dinner: _____
Snacks: _____

GROUP	FRUITS	VEGETABLES	GRAINS	MEAT & BEANS	MILK	OILS
Goal Amount						
Estimate Your Total						
Total Calories						

Physical Activity: _____ Spiritual Activity: _____
Steps/Miles/Minutes: _____ My Emotions Today: ❑ Happy ❑ Sad ❑ Stressed

---

Day/Date:

Breakfast: _____
Lunch: _____
Dinner: _____
Snacks: _____

GROUP	FRUITS	VEGETABLES	GRAINS	MEAT & BEANS	MILK	OILS
Goal Amount						
Estimate Your Total						
Total Calories						

Physical Activity: _____ Spiritual Activity: _____
Steps/Miles/Minutes: _____ My Emotions Today: ❑ Happy ❑ Sad ❑ Stressed

---

Day/Date:

Breakfast: _____
Lunch: _____
Dinner: _____
Snacks: _____

GROUP	FRUITS	VEGETABLES	GRAINS	MEAT & BEANS	MILK	OILS
Goal Amount						
Estimate Your Total						
Total Calories						

Physical Activity: _____ Spiritual Activity: _____
Steps/Miles/Minutes: _____ My Emotions Today: ❑ Happy ❑ Sad ❑ Stressed

Live It Tracker

Name: _____ Date: _____ Week #: _____

Loss/gain _____ lbs.   Calorie Range: _____   My food goal for the week: _____

Activity Level: None, < 30 min/day, 30-60 min/day, 60+ min/day   My activity goal for the week: _____

My spiritual goal for the week: _____

Group	Daily Calories							
	1300-1400	1500-1600	1700-1800	1900-2000	2100-2200	2300-2400	2500-2600	2700-2800
Fruits	1.5-2 c.	1.5-2 c.	1.5-2 c.	2-2.5 c.	2-2.5 c.	2.5-3.5 c.	3.5-4.5 c.	3.5-4.5 c.
Vegetables	1.5-2 c.	2-2.5 c.	2.5-3 c.	2.5-3 c.	3-3.5 c.	3.5-4.5 c.	4.5-5 c.	4.5-5 c.
Grains	5 oz-eq.	5-6 oz-eq.	6-7 oz-eq.	6-7 oz-eq.	7-8 oz-eq.	8-9 oz-eq.	9-10 oz-eq.	10-11 oz-eq.
Meat & Beans	4 oz-eq.	5 oz-eq.	5-5.5 oz-eq.	5.5-6.5 oz-eq.	6.5-7 oz-eq.	7-7.5 oz-eq.	7-7.5 oz-eq.	7.5-8 oz-eq.
Milk	2-3 c.	3 c.	3 c.	3 c.	3 c.	3 c.	3 c.	3 c.
Healthy Oils	4 tsp.	5 tsp.	5 tsp.	6 tsp.	6 tsp.	7 tsp.	8 tsp.	8 tsp.

Day/Date:

Breakfast: _____
Lunch: _____
Dinner: _____
Snacks: _____

GROUP	FRUITS	VEGETABLES	GRAINS	MEAT & BEANS	MILK	OILS
Goal Amount						
Estimate Your Total						
Total Calories						

Physical Activity: _____   Spiritual Activity: _____
Steps/Miles/Minutes: _____   My Emotions Today: ❏ Happy   ❏ Sad   ❏ Stressed

Day/Date:

Breakfast: _____
Lunch: _____
Dinner: _____
Snacks: _____

GROUP	FRUITS	VEGETABLES	GRAINS	MEAT & BEANS	MILK	OILS
Goal Amount						
Estimate Your Total						
Total Calories						

Physical Activity: _____   Spiritual Activity: _____
Steps/Miles/Minutes: _____   My Emotions Today: ❏ Happy   ❏ Sad   ❏ Stressed

Day/Date:

Breakfast: _____
Lunch: _____
Dinner: _____
Snacks: _____

GROUP	FRUITS	VEGETABLES	GRAINS	MEAT & BEANS	MILK	OILS
Goal Amount						
Estimate Your Total						
Total Calories						

Physical Activity: _____   Spiritual Activity: _____
Steps/Miles/Minutes: _____   My Emotions Today: ❏ Happy   ❏ Sad   ❏ Stressed

Day/Date:

Breakfast: _____
Lunch: _____
Dinner: _____
Snacks: _____

GROUP	FRUITS	VEGETABLES	GRAINS	MEAT & BEANS	MILK	OILS
Goal Amount						
Estimate Your Total						
Total Calories						

Physical Activity: _____ Spiritual Activity: _____
Steps/Miles/Minutes: _____ My Emotions Today: ❑ Happy ❑ Sad ❑ Stressed

---

Day/Date:

Breakfast: _____
Lunch: _____
Dinner: _____
Snacks: _____

GROUP	FRUITS	VEGETABLES	GRAINS	MEAT & BEANS	MILK	OILS
Goal Amount						
Estimate Your Total						
Total Calories						

Physical Activity: _____ Spiritual Activity: _____
Steps/Miles/Minutes: _____ My Emotions Today: ❑ Happy ❑ Sad ❑ Stressed

---

Day/Date:

Breakfast: _____
Lunch: _____
Dinner: _____
Snacks: _____

GROUP	FRUITS	VEGETABLES	GRAINS	MEAT & BEANS	MILK	OILS
Goal Amount						
Estimate Your Total						
Total Calories						

Physical Activity: _____ Spiritual Activity: _____
Steps/Miles/Minutes: _____ My Emotions Today: ❑ Happy ❑ Sad ❑ Stressed

---

Day/Date:

Breakfast: _____
Lunch: _____
Dinner: _____
Snacks: _____

GROUP	FRUITS	VEGETABLES	GRAINS	MEAT & BEANS	MILK	OILS
Goal Amount						
Estimate Your Total						
Total Calories						

Physical Activity: _____ Spiritual Activity: _____
Steps/Miles/Minutes: _____ My Emotions Today: ❑ Happy ❑ Sad ❑ Stressed

Live It Tracker

Name: _____ Date: _____ Week #: _____

Loss/gain _____ lbs.   Calorie Range: _____ My food goal for the week: _____

_____

Activity Level: None, < 30 min/day, 30-60 min/day, 60+ min/day   My activity goal for the week: _____

My spiritual goal for the week: _____

Group	Daily Calories							
	1300-1400	1500-1600	1700-1800	1900-2000	2100-2200	2300-2400	2500-2600	2700-2800
Fruits	1.5-2 c.	1.5-2 c.	1.5-2 c.	2-2.5 c.	2-2.5 c.	2.5-3.5 c.	3.5-4.5 c.	3.5-4.5 c.
Vegetables	1.5-2 c.	2-2.5 c.	2.5-3 c.	2.5-3 c.	3-3.5 c.	3.5-4.5 c.	4.5-5 c.	4.5-5 c.
Grains	5 oz-eq.	5-6 oz-eq.	6-7 oz-eq.	6-7 oz-eq.	7-8 oz-eq.	8-9 oz-eq.	9-10 oz-eq.	10-11 oz-eq.
Meat & Beans	4 oz-eq.	5 oz-eq.	5-5.5 oz-eq.	5.5-6.5 oz-eq.	6.5-7 oz-eq.	7-7.5 oz-eq.	7-7.5 oz-eq.	7.5-8 oz-eq.
Milk	2-3 c.	3 c.	3 c.	3 c.	3 c.	3 c.	3 c.	3 c.
Healthy Oils	4 tsp.	5 tsp.	5 tsp.	6 tsp.	6 tsp.	7 tsp.	8 tsp.	8 tsp.

Day/Date:

Breakfast: _____
Lunch: _____
Dinner: _____
Snacks: _____

GROUP	FRUITS	VEGETABLES	GRAINS	MEAT & BEANS	MILK	OILS
Goal Amount						
Estimate Your Total						
Total Calories						

Physical Activity: _____   Spiritual Activity: _____
Steps/Miles/Minutes: _____   My Emotions Today: ❏ Happy ❏ Sad ❏ Stressed

Day/Date:

Breakfast: _____
Lunch: _____
Dinner: _____
Snacks: _____

GROUP	FRUITS	VEGETABLES	GRAINS	MEAT & BEANS	MILK	OILS
Goal Amount						
Estimate Your Total						
Total Calories						

Physical Activity: _____   Spiritual Activity: _____
Steps/Miles/Minutes: _____   My Emotions Today: ❏ Happy ❏ Sad ❏ Stressed

Day/Date:

Breakfast: _____
Lunch: _____
Dinner: _____
Snacks: _____

GROUP	FRUITS	VEGETABLES	GRAINS	MEAT & BEANS	MILK	OILS
Goal Amount						
Estimate Your Total						
Total Calories						

Physical Activity: _____   Spiritual Activity: _____
Steps/Miles/Minutes: _____   My Emotions Today: ❏ Happy ❏ Sad ❏ Stressed

Breakfast: _____
Lunch: _____
Dinner: _____
Snacks: _____

GROUP	FRUITS	VEGETABLES	GRAINS	MEAT & BEANS	MILK	OILS
Goal Amount						
Estimate Your Total						
Total Calories						

Physical Activity: _____   Spiritual Activity: _____
Steps/Miles/Minutes: _____   My Emotions Today: ❏ Happy ❏ Sad ❏ Stressed

Breakfast: _____
Lunch: _____
Dinner: _____
Snacks: _____

GROUP	FRUITS	VEGETABLES	GRAINS	MEAT & BEANS	MILK	OILS
Goal Amount						
Estimate Your Total						
Total Calories						

Physical Activity: _____   Spiritual Activity: _____
Steps/Miles/Minutes: _____   My Emotions Today: ❏ Happy ❏ Sad ❏ Stressed

Breakfast: _____
Lunch: _____
Dinner: _____
Snacks: _____

GROUP	FRUITS	VEGETABLES	GRAINS	MEAT & BEANS	MILK	OILS
Goal Amount						
Estimate Your Total						
Total Calories						

Physical Activity: _____   Spiritual Activity: _____
Steps/Miles/Minutes: _____   My Emotions Today: ❏ Happy ❏ Sad ❏ Stressed

Breakfast: _____
Lunch: _____
Dinner: _____
Snacks: _____

GROUP	FRUITS	VEGETABLES	GRAINS	MEAT & BEANS	MILK	OILS
Goal Amount						
Estimate Your Total						
Total Calories						

Physical Activity: _____   Spiritual Activity: _____
Steps/Miles/Minutes: _____   My Emotions Today: ❏ Happy ❏ Sad ❏ Stressed

Live It Tracker

Name: _____ Date: _____ Week #: _____

Loss/gain _____ lbs.   Calorie Range: _____   My food goal for the week: _____

Activity Level: None, < 30 min/day, 30-60 min/day, 60+ min/day   My activity goal for the week: _____

My spiritual goal for the week: _____

Group	Daily Calories							
	1300-1400	1500-1600	1700-1800	1900-2000	2100-2200	2300-2400	2500-2600	2700-2800
Fruits	1.5-2 c.	1.5-2 c.	1.5-2 c.	2-2.5 c.	2-2.5 c.	2.5-3.5 c.	3.5-4.5 c	3.5-4.5 c.
Vegetables	1.5-2 c.	2-2.5 c.	2.5-3 c.	2.5-3 c.	3-3.5 c.	3.5-4.5 c.	4.5-5 c.	4.5-5 c.
Grains	5 oz-eq.	5-6 oz-eq.	6-7 oz-eq.	6-7 oz-eq.	7-8 oz-eq.	8-9 oz-eq.	9-10 oz-eq.	10-11 oz-eq.
Meat & Beans	4 oz-eq.	5 oz-eq.	5-5.5 oz-eq.	5.5-6.5 oz-eq.	6.5-7 oz-eq.	7-7.5 oz-eq.	7-7.5 oz-eq.	7.5-8 oz-eq.
Milk	2-3 c.	3 c.	3 c.	3 c.	3 c.	3 c.	3 c.	3 c.
Healthy Oils	4 tsp.	5 tsp.	5 tsp.	6 tsp.	6 tsp.	7 tsp.	8 tsp.	8 tsp.

Day/Date:

Breakfast: _____
Lunch: _____
Dinner: _____
Snacks: _____

GROUP	FRUITS	VEGETABLES	GRAINS	MEAT & BEANS	MILK	OILS
Goal Amount						
Estimate Your Total						
Total Calories						

Physical Activity: _____   Spiritual Activity: _____
Steps/Miles/Minutes: _____   My Emotions Today: ❑ Happy   ❑ Sad   ❑ Stressed

Day/Date:

Breakfast: _____
Lunch: _____
Dinner: _____
Snacks: _____

GROUP	FRUITS	VEGETABLES	GRAINS	MEAT & BEANS	MILK	OILS
Goal Amount						
Estimate Your Total						
Total Calories						

Physical Activity: _____   Spiritual Activity: _____
Steps/Miles/Minutes: _____   My Emotions Today: ❑ Happy   ❑ Sad   ❑ Stressed

Day/Date:

Breakfast: _____
Lunch: _____
Dinner: _____
Snacks: _____

GROUP	FRUITS	VEGETABLES	GRAINS	MEAT & BEANS	MILK	OILS
Goal Amount						
Estimate Your Total						
Total Calories						

Physical Activity: _____   Spiritual Activity: _____
Steps/Miles/Minutes: _____   My Emotions Today: ❑ Happy   ❑ Sad   ❑ Stressed

Day/Date:

Breakfast: _____
Lunch: _____
Dinner: _____
Snacks: _____

GROUP	FRUITS	VEGETABLES	GRAINS	MEAT & BEANS	MILK	OILS
Goal Amount						
Estimate Your Total						
Total Calories						

Physical Activity: _____ Spiritual Activity: _____

Steps/Miles/Minutes: _____ My Emotions Today: ❑ Happy ❑ Sad ❑ Stressed

---

Day/Date:

Breakfast: _____
Lunch: _____
Dinner: _____
Snacks: _____

GROUP	FRUITS	VEGETABLES	GRAINS	MEAT & BEANS	MILK	OILS
Goal Amount						
Estimate Your Total						
Total Calories						

Physical Activity: _____ Spiritual Activity: _____

Steps/Miles/Minutes: _____ My Emotions Today: ❑ Happy ❑ Sad ❑ Stressed

---

Day/Date:

Breakfast: _____
Lunch: _____
Dinner: _____
Snacks: _____

GROUP	FRUITS	VEGETABLES	GRAINS	MEAT & BEANS	MILK	OILS
Goal Amount						
Estimate Your Total						
Total Calories						

Physical Activity: _____ Spiritual Activity: _____

Steps/Miles/Minutes: _____ My Emotions Today: ❑ Happy ❑ Sad ❑ Stressed

---

Day/Date:

Breakfast: _____
Lunch: _____
Dinner: _____
Snacks: _____

GROUP	FRUITS	VEGETABLES	GRAINS	MEAT & BEANS	MILK	OILS
Goal Amount						
Estimate Your Total						
Total Calories						

Physical Activity: _____ Spiritual Activity: _____

Steps/Miles/Minutes: _____ My Emotions Today: ❑ Happy ❑ Sad ❑ Stressed

Live It Tracker

Name: _____ Date: _____ Week #: _____

Loss/gain _____ lbs. Calorie Range: _____ My food goal for the week: _____

_____

Activity Level: None, < 30 min/day, 30-60 min/day, 60+ min/day   My activity goal for the week: _____

My spiritual goal for the week: _____

Group	Daily Calories							
	1300-1400	1500-1600	1700-1800	1900-2000	2100-2200	2300-2400	2500-2600	2700-2800
Fruits	1.5-2 c.	1.5-2 c.	1.5-2 c.	2-2.5 c.	2-2.5 c.	2.5-3.5 c.	3.5-4.5 c.	3.5-4.5 c.
Vegetables	1.5-2 c.	2-2.5 c.	2.5-3 c.	2.5-3 c.	3-3.5 c.	3.5-4.5 c.	4.5-5 c.	4.5-5 c.
Grains	5 oz-eq.	5-6 oz-eq.	6-7 oz-eq.	6-7 oz-eq.	7-8 oz-eq.	8-9 oz-eq.	9-10 oz-eq.	10-11 oz-eq.
Meat & Beans	4 oz-eq.	5 oz-eq.	5-5.5 oz-eq.	5.5-6.5 oz-eq.	6.5-7 oz-eq.	7-7.5 oz-eq.	7-7.5 oz-eq.	7.5-8 oz-eq.
Milk	2-3 c.	3 c.	3 c.	3 c.	3 c.	3 c.	3 c.	3 c.
Healthy Oils	4 tsp.	5 tsp.	5 tsp.	6 tsp.	6 tsp.	7 tsp.	8 tsp.	8 tsp.

Day/Date:

Breakfast: _____
Lunch: _____
Dinner: _____
Snacks: _____

GROUP	FRUITS	VEGETABLES	GRAINS	MEAT & BEANS	MILK	OILS
Goal Amount						
Estimate Your Total						
Total Calories						

Physical Activity: _____ Spiritual Activity: _____
Steps/Miles/Minutes: _____ My Emotions Today: ❑ Happy ❑ Sad ❑ Stressed

Day/Date:

Breakfast: _____
Lunch: _____
Dinner: _____
Snacks: _____

GROUP	FRUITS	VEGETABLES	GRAINS	MEAT & BEANS	MILK	OILS
Goal Amount						
Estimate Your Total						
Total Calories						

Physical Activity: _____ Spiritual Activity: _____
Steps/Miles/Minutes: _____ My Emotions Today: ❑ Happy ❑ Sad ❑ Stressed

Day/Date:

Breakfast: _____
Lunch: _____
Dinner: _____
Snacks: _____

GROUP	FRUITS	VEGETABLES	GRAINS	MEAT & BEANS	MILK	OILS
Goal Amount						
Estimate Your Total						
Total Calories						

Physical Activity: _____ Spiritual Activity: _____
Steps/Miles/Minutes: _____ My Emotions Today: ❑ Happy ❑ Sad ❑ Stressed

Day/Date:

Breakfast: _____

Lunch: _____

Dinner: _____

Snacks: _____

GROUP	FRUITS	VEGETABLES	GRAINS	MEAT & BEANS	MILK	OILS
Goal Amount						
Estimate Your Total						
Total Calories						

Physical Activity: _____   Spiritual Activity: _____

Steps/Miles/Minutes: _____   My Emotions Today: ❏ Happy   ❏ Sad   ❏ Stressed

Day/Date:

Breakfast: _____

Lunch: _____

Dinner: _____

Snacks: _____

GROUP	FRUITS	VEGETABLES	GRAINS	MEAT & BEANS	MILK	OILS
Goal Amount						
Estimate Your Total						
Total Calories						

Physical Activity: _____   Spiritual Activity: _____

Steps/Miles/Minutes: _____   My Emotions Today: ❏ Happy   ❏ Sad   ❏ Stressed

Day/Date:

Breakfast: _____

Lunch: _____

Dinner: _____

Snacks: _____

GROUP	FRUITS	VEGETABLES	GRAINS	MEAT & BEANS	MILK	OILS
Goal Amount						
Estimate Your Total						
Total Calories						

Physical Activity: _____   Spiritual Activity: _____

Steps/Miles/Minutes: _____   My Emotions Today: ❏ Happy   ❏ Sad   ❏ Stressed

Day/Date:

Breakfast: _____

Lunch: _____

Dinner: _____

Snacks: _____

GROUP	FRUITS	VEGETABLES	GRAINS	MEAT & BEANS	MILK	OILS
Goal Amount						
Estimate Your Total						
Total Calories						

Physical Activity: _____   Spiritual Activity: _____

Steps/Miles/Minutes: _____   My Emotions Today: ❏ Happy   ❏ Sad   ❏ Stressed

Live It Tracker

Name: _____ Date: _____ Week #: _____

Loss/gain _____ lbs. Calorie Range: _____ My food goal for the week: _____

_____

Activity Level: None, < 30 min/day, 30-60 min/day, 60+ min/day My activity goal for the week: _____

My spiritual goal for the week: _____

Group	Daily Calories							
	1300-1400	1500-1600	1700-1800	1900-2000	2100-2200	2300-2400	2500-2600	2700-2800
Fruits	1.5-2 c.	1.5-2 c.	1.5-2 c.	2-2.5 c.	2-2.5 c.	2.5-3.5 c.	3.5-4.5 c.	3.5-4.5 c.
Vegetables	1.5-2 c.	2-2.5 c.	2.5-3 c.	2.5-3 c.	3-3.5 c.	3.5-4.5 c.	4.5-5 c.	4.5-5 c.
Grains	5 oz-eq.	5-6 oz-eq.	6-7 oz-eq.	6-7 oz-eq.	7-8 oz-eq.	8-9 oz-eq.	9-10 oz-eq.	10-11 oz-eq.
Meat & Beans	4 oz-eq.	5 oz-eq.	5-5.5 oz-eq.	5.5-6.5 oz-eq.	6.5-7 oz-eq.	7-7.5 oz-eq.	7-7.5 oz-eq.	7.5-8 oz-eq.
Milk	2-3 c.	3 c.	3 c.	3 c.	3 c.	3 c.	3 c.	3 c.
Healthy Oils	4 tsp.	5 tsp.	5 tsp.	6 tsp.	6 tsp.	7 tsp.	8 tsp.	8 tsp.

Day/Date:

Breakfast: _____
Lunch: _____
Dinner: _____
Snacks: _____

GROUP	FRUITS	VEGETABLES	GRAINS	MEAT & BEANS	MILK	OILS
Goal Amount						
Estimate Your Total						
Total Calories						

Physical Activity: _____ Spiritual Activity: _____
Steps/Miles/Minutes: _____ My Emotions Today: ❑ Happy   ❑ Sad   ❑ Stressed

Day/Date:

Breakfast: _____
Lunch: _____
Dinner: _____
Snacks: _____

GROUP	FRUITS	VEGETABLES	GRAINS	MEAT & BEANS	MILK	OILS
Goal Amount						
Estimate Your Total						
Total Calories						

Physical Activity: _____ Spiritual Activity: _____
Steps/Miles/Minutes: _____ My Emotions Today: ❑ Happy   ❑ Sad   ❑ Stressed

Day/Date:

Breakfast: _____
Lunch: _____
Dinner: _____
Snacks: _____

GROUP	FRUITS	VEGETABLES	GRAINS	MEAT & BEANS	MILK	OILS
Goal Amount						
Estimate Your Total						
Total Calories						

Physical Activity: _____ Spiritual Activity: _____
Steps/Miles/Minutes: _____ My Emotions Today: ❑ Happy   ❑ Sad   ❑ Stressed

Breakfast: _____

Lunch: _____

Dinner: _____

Snacks: _____

GROUP	FRUITS	VEGETABLES	GRAINS	MEAT & BEANS	MILK	OILS
Goal Amount						
Estimate Your Total						
Total Calories						

Physical Activity: _____   **Spiritual Activity:** _____

Steps/Miles/Minutes: _____   My Emotions Today: ❑ Happy   ❑ Sad   ❑ Stressed

Day/Date:

Breakfast: _____

Lunch: _____

Dinner: _____

Snacks: _____

GROUP	FRUITS	VEGETABLES	GRAINS	MEAT & BEANS	MILK	OILS
Goal Amount						
Estimate Your Total						
Total Calories						

Physical Activity: _____   **Spiritual Activity:** _____

Steps/Miles/Minutes: _____   My Emotions Today: ❑ Happy   ❑ Sad   ❑ Stressed

Day/Date:

Breakfast: _____

Lunch: _____

Dinner: _____

Snacks: _____

GROUP	FRUITS	VEGETABLES	GRAINS	MEAT & BEANS	MILK	OILS
Goal Amount						
Estimate Your Total						
Total Calories						

Physical Activity: _____   **Spiritual Activity:** _____

Steps/Miles/Minutes: _____   My Emotions Today: ❑ Happy   ❑ Sad   ❑ Stressed

Day/Date:

Breakfast: _____

Lunch: _____

Dinner: _____

Snacks: _____

GROUP	FRUITS	VEGETABLES	GRAINS	MEAT & BEANS	MILK	OILS
Goal Amount						
Estimate Your Total						
Total Calories						

Physical Activity: _____   **Spiritual Activity:** _____

Steps/Miles/Minutes: _____   My Emotions Today: ❑ Happy   ❑ Sad   ❑ Stressed

Day/Date:

Live It Tracker

Name: _____ Date: _____ Week #: _____

Loss/gain _____ lbs. Calorie Range: _____ My food goal for the week: _____

Activity Level: None, < 30 min/day, 30-60 min/day, 60+ min/day   My activity goal for the week: _____

My spiritual goal for the week: _____

Group	Daily Calories							
	1300-1400	1500-1600	1700-1800	1900-2000	2100-2200	2300-2400	2500-2600	2700-2800
Fruits	1.5-2 c.	1.5-2 c.	1.5-2 c.	2-2.5 c.	2-2.5 c.	2.5-3.5 c.	3.5-4.5 c.	3.5-4.5 c.
Vegetables	1.5-2 c.	2-2.5 c.	2.5-3 c.	2.5-3 c.	3-3.5 c.	3.5-4.5 c.	4.5-5 c.	4.5-5 c.
Grains	5 oz-eq.	5-6 oz-eq.	6-7 oz-eq.	6-7 oz-eq.	7-8 oz-eq.	8-9 oz-eq.	9-10 oz-eq.	10-11 oz-eq.
Meat & Beans	4 oz-eq.	5 oz-eq.	5-5.5 oz-eq.	5.5-6.5 oz-eq.	6.5-7 oz-eq.	7-7.5 oz-eq.	7-7.5 oz-eq.	7.5-8 oz-eq.
Milk	2-3 c.	3 c.	3 c.	3 c.	3 c.	3 c.	3 c.	3 c.
Healthy Oils	4 tsp.	5 tsp.	5 tsp.	6 tsp.	6 tsp.	7 tsp.	8 tsp.	8 tsp.

Day/Date:

Breakfast: _____
Lunch: _____
Dinner: _____
Snacks: _____

GROUP	FRUITS	VEGETABLES	GRAINS	MEAT & BEANS	MILK	OILS
Goal Amount						
Estimate Your Total						
Total Calories						

Physical Activity: _____ Spiritual Activity: _____
Steps/Miles/Minutes: _____ My Emotions Today: ❏ Happy ❏ Sad ❏ Stressed

Day/Date:

Breakfast: _____
Lunch: _____
Dinner: _____
Snacks: _____

GROUP	FRUITS	VEGETABLES	GRAINS	MEAT & BEANS	MILK	OILS
Goal Amount						
Estimate Your Total						
Total Calories						

Physical Activity: _____ Spiritual Activity: _____
Steps/Miles/Minutes: _____ My Emotions Today: ❏ Happy ❏ Sad ❏ Stressed

Day/Date:

Breakfast: _____
Lunch: _____
Dinner: _____
Snacks: _____

GROUP	FRUITS	VEGETABLES	GRAINS	MEAT & BEANS	MILK	OILS
Goal Amount						
Estimate Your Total						
Total Calories						

Physical Activity: _____ Spiritual Activity: _____
Steps/Miles/Minutes: _____ My Emotions Today: ❏ Happy ❏ Sad ❏ Stressed

Day/Date:

Breakfast: _____
Lunch: _____
Dinner: _____
Snacks: _____

GROUP	FRUITS	VEGETABLES	GRAINS	MEAT & BEANS	MILK	OILS
Goal Amount						
Estimate Your Total						
Total Calories						

Physical Activity: _____ Spiritual Activity: _____

Steps/Miles/Minutes: _____ My Emotions Today: ❑ Happy ❑ Sad ❑ Stressed

---

Day/Date:

Breakfast: _____
Lunch: _____
Dinner: _____
Snacks: _____

GROUP	FRUITS	VEGETABLES	GRAINS	MEAT & BEANS	MILK	OILS
Goal Amount						
Estimate Your Total						
Total Calories						

Physical Activity: _____ Spiritual Activity: _____

Steps/Miles/Minutes: _____ My Emotions Today: ❑ Happy ❑ Sad ❑ Stressed

---

Day/Date:

Breakfast: _____
Lunch: _____
Dinner: _____
Snacks: _____

GROUP	FRUITS	VEGETABLES	GRAINS	MEAT & BEANS	MILK	OILS
Goal Amount						
Estimate Your Total						
Total Calories						

Physical Activity: _____ Spiritual Activity: _____

Steps/Miles/Minutes: _____ My Emotions Today: ❑ Happy ❑ Sad ❑ Stressed

---

Day/Date:

Breakfast: _____
Lunch: _____
Dinner: _____
Snacks: _____

GROUP	FRUITS	VEGETABLES	GRAINS	MEAT & BEANS	MILK	OILS
Goal Amount						
Estimate Your Total						
Total Calories						

Physical Activity: _____ Spiritual Activity: _____

Steps/Miles/Minutes: _____ My Emotions Today: ❑ Happy ❑ Sad ❑ Stressed

Live It Tracker

Name: _____ Date: _____ Week #: _____

Loss/gain _____ lbs.   Calorie Range: _____   My food goal for the week: _____

_____

Activity Level: None, < 30 min/day, 30-60 min/day, 60+ min/day   My activity goal for the week: _____

My spiritual goal for the week: _____

Group	Daily Calories							
	1300-1400	1500-1600	1700-1800	1900-2000	2100-2200	2300-2400	2500-2600	2700-2800
Fruits	1.5-2 c.	1.5-2 c.	1.5-2 c.	2-2.5 c.	2-2.5 c.	2.5-3.5 c.	3.5-4.5 c.	3.5-4.5 c.
Vegetables	1.5-2 c.	2-2.5 c.	2.5-3 c.	2.5-3 c.	3-3.5 c.	3.5-4.5 c.	4.5-5 c.	4.5-5 c.
Grains	5 oz-eq.	5-6 oz-eq.	6-7 oz-eq.	6-7 oz-eq.	7-8 oz-eq.	8-9 oz-eq.	9-10 oz-eq.	10-11 oz-eq.
Meat & Beans	4 oz-eq.	5 oz-eq.	5-5.5 oz-eq.	5.5-6.5 oz-eq.	6.5-7 oz-eq.	7-7.5 oz-eq.	7-7.5 oz-eq.	7.5-8 oz-eq.
Milk	2-3 c.	3 c.	3 c.	3 c.	3 c.	3 c.	3 c.	3 c.
Healthy Oils	4 tsp.	5 tsp.	5 tsp.	6 tsp.	6 tsp.	7 tsp.	8 tsp.	8 tsp.

Day/Date:

Breakfast: _____
Lunch: _____
Dinner: _____
Snacks: _____

GROUP	FRUITS	VEGETABLES	GRAINS	MEAT & BEANS	MILK	OILS
Goal Amount						
Estimate Your Total						
Total Calories						

Physical Activity: _____   Spiritual Activity: _____
Steps/Miles/Minutes: _____   My Emotions Today: ❑ Happy ❑ Sad ❑ Stressed

Day/Date:

Breakfast: _____
Lunch: _____
Dinner: _____
Snacks: _____

GROUP	FRUITS	VEGETABLES	GRAINS	MEAT & BEANS	MILK	OILS
Goal Amount						
Estimate Your Total						
Total Calories						

Physical Activity: _____   Spiritual Activity: _____
Steps/Miles/Minutes: _____   My Emotions Today: ❑ Happy ❑ Sad ❑ Stressed

Day/Date:

Breakfast: _____
Lunch: _____
Dinner: _____
Snacks: _____

GROUP	FRUITS	VEGETABLES	GRAINS	MEAT & BEANS	MILK	OILS
Goal Amount						
Estimate Your Total						
Total Calories						

Physical Activity: _____   Spiritual Activity: _____
Steps/Miles/Minutes: _____   My Emotions Today: ❑ Happy ❑ Sad ❑ Stressed

Day/Date:

Breakfast: _____
Lunch: _____
Dinner: _____
Snacks: _____

GROUP	FRUITS	VEGETABLES	GRAINS	MEAT & BEANS	MILK	OILS
Goal Amount						
Estimate Your Total						
Total Calories						

Physical Activity: _____ Spiritual Activity: _____
Steps/Miles/Minutes: _____ My Emotions Today: ❑ Happy ❑ Sad ❑ Stressed

---

Day/Date:

Breakfast: _____
Lunch: _____
Dinner: _____
Snacks: _____

GROUP	FRUITS	VEGETABLES	GRAINS	MEAT & BEANS	MILK	OILS
Goal Amount						
Estimate Your Total						
Total Calories						

Physical Activity: _____ Spiritual Activity: _____
Steps/Miles/Minutes: _____ My Emotions Today: ❑ Happy ❑ Sad ❑ Stressed

---

Day/Date:

Breakfast: _____
Lunch: _____
Dinner: _____
Snacks: _____

GROUP	FRUITS	VEGETABLES	GRAINS	MEAT & BEANS	MILK	OILS
Goal Amount						
Estimate Your Total						
Total Calories						

Physical Activity: _____ Spiritual Activity: _____
Steps/Miles/Minutes: _____ My Emotions Today: ❑ Happy ❑ Sad ❑ Stressed

---

Day/Date:

Breakfast: _____
Lunch: _____
Dinner: _____
Snacks: _____

GROUP	FRUITS	VEGETABLES	GRAINS	MEAT & BEANS	MILK	OILS
Goal Amount						
Estimate Your Total						
Total Calories						

Physical Activity: _____ Spiritual Activity: _____
Steps/Miles/Minutes: _____ My Emotions Today: ❑ Happy ❑ Sad ❑ Stressed

Live It Tracker

Name: _____ Date: _____ Week #: _____

Loss/gain _____ lbs.   Calorie Range: _____   My food goal for the week: _____

Activity Level: None, < 30 min/day, 30-60 min/day, 60+ min/day   My activity goal for the week: _____

My spiritual goal for the week: _____

Group	Daily Calories							
	1300-1400	1500-1600	1700-1800	1900-2000	2100-2200	2300-2400	2500-2600	2700-2800
Fruits	1.5-2 c.	1.5-2 c.	1.5-2 c.	2-2.5 c.	2-2.5 c.	2.5-3.5 c.	3.5-4.5 c.	3.5-4.5 c.
Vegetables	1.5-2 c.	2-2.5 c.	2.5-3 c.	2.5-3 c.	3-3.5 c.	3.5-4.5 c.	4.5-5 c.	4.5-5 c.
Grains	5 oz-eq.	5-6 oz-eq.	6-7 oz-eq.	6-7 oz-eq.	7-8 oz-eq.	8-9 oz-eq.	9-10 oz-eq.	10-11 oz-eq.
Meat & Beans	4 oz-eq.	5 oz-eq.	5-5.5 oz-eq.	5.5-6.5 oz-eq.	6.5-7 oz-eq.	7-7.5 oz-eq.	7-7.5 oz-eq.	7.5-8 oz-eq.
Milk	2-3 c.	3 c.	3 c.	3 c.	3 c.	3 c.	3 c.	3 c.
Healthy Oils	4 tsp.	5 tsp.	5 tsp.	6 tsp.	6 tsp.	7 tsp.	8 tsp.	8 tsp.

Day/Date:

Breakfast: _____

Lunch: _____

Dinner: _____

Snacks: _____

GROUP	FRUITS	VEGETABLES	GRAINS	MEAT & BEANS	MILK	OILS
Goal Amount						
Estimate Your Total						
Total Calories						

Physical Activity: _____   Spiritual Activity: _____

Steps/Miles/Minutes: _____   My Emotions Today: ❑ Happy   ❑ Sad   ❑ Stressed

Day/Date:

Breakfast: _____

Lunch: _____

Dinner: _____

Snacks: _____

GROUP	FRUITS	VEGETABLES	GRAINS	MEAT & BEANS	MILK	OILS
Goal Amount						
Estimate Your Total						
Total Calories						

Physical Activity: _____   Spiritual Activity: _____

Steps/Miles/Minutes: _____   My Emotions Today: ❑ Happy   ❑ Sad   ❑ Stressed

Day/Date:

Breakfast: _____

Lunch: _____

Dinner: _____

Snacks: _____

GROUP	FRUITS	VEGETABLES	GRAINS	MEAT & BEANS	MILK	OILS
Goal Amount						
Estimate Your Total						
Total Calories						

Physical Activity: _____   Spiritual Activity: _____

Steps/Miles/Minutes: _____   My Emotions Today: ❑ Happy   ❑ Sad   ❑ Stressed

Day/Date:

Breakfast: _____
Lunch: _____
Dinner: _____
Snacks: _____

GROUP	FRUITS	VEGETABLES	GRAINS	MEAT & BEANS	MILK	OILS
Goal Amount						
Estimate Your Total						
Total Calories						

Physical Activity: _____   Spiritual Activity: _____
Steps/Miles/Minutes: _____   My Emotions Today: ❑ Happy ❑ Sad ❑ Stressed

Day/Date:

Breakfast: _____
Lunch: _____
Dinner: _____
Snacks: _____

GROUP	FRUITS	VEGETABLES	GRAINS	MEAT & BEANS	MILK	OILS
Goal Amount						
Estimate Your Total						
Total Calories						

Physical Activity: _____   Spiritual Activity: _____
Steps/Miles/Minutes: _____   My Emotions Today: ❑ Happy ❑ Sad ❑ Stressed

Day/Date:

Breakfast: _____
Lunch: _____
Dinner: _____
Snacks: _____

GROUP	FRUITS	VEGETABLES	GRAINS	MEAT & BEANS	MILK	OILS
Goal Amount						
Estimate Your Total						
Total Calories						

Physical Activity: _____   Spiritual Activity: _____
Steps/Miles/Minutes: _____   My Emotions Today: ❑ Happy ❑ Sad ❑ Stressed

Day/Date:

Breakfast: _____
Lunch: _____
Dinner: _____
Snacks: _____

GROUP	FRUITS	VEGETABLES	GRAINS	MEAT & BEANS	MILK	OILS
Goal Amount						
Estimate Your Total						
Total Calories						

Physical Activity: _____   Spiritual Activity: _____
Steps/Miles/Minutes: _____   My Emotions Today: ❑ Happy ❑ Sad ❑ Stressed

Live It Tracker

Name: _____ Date: _____ Week #: _____

Loss/gain _____ lbs. Calorie Range: _____ My food goal for the week: _____

_____

Activity Level: None, < 30 min/day, 30-60 min/day, 60+ min/day   My activity goal for the week: _____

My spiritual goal for the week: _____

Group	Daily Calories							
	1300-1400	1500-1600	1700-1800	1900-2000	2100-2200	2300-2400	2500-2600	2700-2800
Fruits	1.5-2 c.	1.5-2 c.	1.5-2 c.	2-2.5 c.	2-2.5 c.	2.5-3.5 c.	3.5-4.5 c.	3.5-4.5 c.
Vegetables	1.5-2 c.	2-2.5 c.	2.5-3 c.	2.5-3 c.	3-3.5 c.	3.5-4.5 c.	4.5-5 c.	4.5-5 c.
Grains	5 oz-eq.	5-6 oz-eq.	6-7 oz-eq.	6-7 oz-eq.	7-8 oz-eq.	8-9 oz-eq.	9-10 oz-eq.	10-11 oz-eq.
Meat & Beans	4 oz-eq.	5 oz-eq.	5-5.5 oz-eq.	5.5-6.5 oz-eq.	6.5-7 oz-eq.	7-7.5 oz-eq.	7-7.5 oz-eq.	7.5-8 oz-eq.
Milk	2-3 c.	3 c.	3 c.	3 c.	3 c.	3 c.	3 c.	3 c.
Healthy Oils	4 tsp.	5 tsp.	5 tsp.	6 tsp.	6 tsp.	7 tsp.	8 tsp.	8 tsp.

Day/Date:

Breakfast: _____

Lunch: _____

Dinner: _____

Snacks: _____

GROUP	FRUITS	VEGETABLES	GRAINS	MEAT & BEANS	MILK	OILS
Goal Amount						
Estimate Your Total						
Total Calories						

Physical Activity: _____ Spiritual Activity: _____

Steps/Miles/Minutes: _____ My Emotions Today: ❏ Happy ❏ Sad ❏ Stressed

Day/Date:

Breakfast: _____

Lunch: _____

Dinner: _____

Snacks: _____

GROUP	FRUITS	VEGETABLES	GRAINS	MEAT & BEANS	MILK	OILS
Goal Amount						
Estimate Your Total						
Total Calories						

Physical Activity: _____ Spiritual Activity: _____

Steps/Miles/Minutes: _____ My Emotions Today: ❏ Happy ❏ Sad ❏ Stressed

Day/Date:

Breakfast: _____

Lunch: _____

Dinner: _____

Snacks: _____

GROUP	FRUITS	VEGETABLES	GRAINS	MEAT & BEANS	MILK	OILS
Goal Amount						
Estimate Your Total						
Total Calories						

Physical Activity: _____ Spiritual Activity: _____

Steps/Miles/Minutes: _____ My Emotions Today: ❏ Happy ❏ Sad ❏ Stressed

Breakfast: _____

Lunch: _____

Dinner: _____

Snacks: _____

GROUP	FRUITS	VEGETABLES	GRAINS	MEAT & BEANS	MILK	OILS
Goal Amount						
Estimate Your Total						
Total Calories						

Physical Activity: _____   **Spiritual Activity:** _____

Steps/Miles/Minutes: _____   **My Emotions Today:** ❑ Happy ❑ Sad ❑ Stressed

---

Breakfast: _____

Lunch: _____

Dinner: _____

Snacks: _____

GROUP	FRUITS	VEGETABLES	GRAINS	MEAT & BEANS	MILK	OILS
Goal Amount						
Estimate Your Total						
Total Calories						

Physical Activity: _____   **Spiritual Activity:** _____

Steps/Miles/Minutes: _____   **My Emotions Today:** ❑ Happy ❑ Sad ❑ Stressed

---

Breakfast: _____

Lunch: _____

Dinner: _____

Snacks: _____

GROUP	FRUITS	VEGETABLES	GRAINS	MEAT & BEANS	MILK	OILS
Goal Amount						
Estimate Your Total						
Total Calories						

Physical Activity: _____   **Spiritual Activity:** _____

Steps/Miles/Minutes: _____   **My Emotions Today:** ❑ Happy ❑ Sad ❑ Stressed

---

Breakfast: _____

Lunch: _____

Dinner: _____

Snacks: _____

GROUP	FRUITS	VEGETABLES	GRAINS	MEAT & BEANS	MILK	OILS
Goal Amount						
Estimate Your Total						
Total Calories						

Physical Activity: _____   **Spiritual Activity:** _____

Steps/Miles/Minutes: _____   **My Emotions Today:** ❑ Happy ❑ Sad ❑ Stressed

Live It Tracker

Name: _____ Date: _____ Week #: _____

Loss/gain _____ lbs.   Calorie Range: _____   My food goal for the week: _____

Activity Level: None, < 30 min/day, 30-60 min/day, 60+ min/day   My activity goal for the week: _____

My spiritual goal for the week: _____

Group	Daily Calories							
	1300-1400	1500-1600	1700-1800	1900-2000	2100-2200	2300-2400	2500-2600	2700-2800
Fruits	1.5-2 c.	1.5-2 c.	1.5-2 c.	2-2.5 c.	2-2.5 c.	2.5-3.5 c.	3.5-4.5 c.	3.5-4.5 c.
Vegetables	1.5-2 c.	2-2.5 c.	2.5-3 c.	2.5-3 c.	3-3.5 c.	3.5-4.5 c.	4.5-5 c.	4.5-5 c.
Grains	5 oz-eq.	5-6 oz-eq.	6-7 oz-eq.	6-7 oz-eq.	7-8 oz-eq.	8-9 oz-eq.	9-10 oz-eq.	10-11 oz-eq.
Meat & Beans	4 oz-eq.	5 oz-eq.	5-5.5 oz-eq.	5.5-6.5 oz-eq.	6.5-7 oz-eq.	7-7.5 oz-eq.	7-7.5 oz-eq.	7.5-8 oz-eq.
Milk	2-3 c.	3 c.	3 c.	3 c.	3 c.	3 c.	3 c.	3 c.
Healthy Oils	4 tsp.	5 tsp.	5 tsp.	6 tsp.	6 tsp.	7 tsp.	8 tsp.	8 tsp.

Day/Date:

Breakfast: _____
Lunch: _____
Dinner: _____
Snacks: _____

GROUP	FRUITS	VEGETABLES	GRAINS	MEAT & BEANS	MILK	OILS
Goal Amount						
Estimate Your Total						
Total Calories						

Physical Activity: _____   Spiritual Activity: _____
Steps/Miles/Minutes: _____   My Emotions Today: ❑ Happy   ❑ Sad   ❑ Stressed

Day/Date:

Breakfast: _____
Lunch: _____
Dinner: _____
Snacks: _____

GROUP	FRUITS	VEGETABLES	GRAINS	MEAT & BEANS	MILK	OILS
Goal Amount						
Estimate Your Total						
Total Calories						

Physical Activity: _____   Spiritual Activity: _____
Steps/Miles/Minutes: _____   My Emotions Today: ❑ Happy   ❑ Sad   ❑ Stressed

Day/Date:

Breakfast: _____
Lunch: _____
Dinner: _____
Snacks: _____

GROUP	FRUITS	VEGETABLES	GRAINS	MEAT & BEANS	MILK	OILS
Goal Amount						
Estimate Your Total						
Total Calories						

Physical Activity: _____   Spiritual Activity: _____
Steps/Miles/Minutes: _____   My Emotions Today: ❑ Happy   ❑ Sad   ❑ Stressed

Breakfast: _____

Lunch: _____

Dinner: _____

Snacks: _____

GROUP	FRUITS	VEGETABLES	GRAINS	MEAT & BEANS	MILK	OILS
Goal Amount						
Estimate Your Total						
Total Calories						

Physical Activity: _____

Steps/Miles/Minutes: _____

Spiritual Activity: _____

My Emotions Today: ❏ Happy ❏ Sad ❏ Stressed

Day/Date:

Breakfast: _____

Lunch: _____

Dinner: _____

Snacks: _____

GROUP	FRUITS	VEGETABLES	GRAINS	MEAT & BEANS	MILK	OILS
Goal Amount						
Estimate Your Total						
Total Calories						

Physical Activity: _____

Steps/Miles/Minutes: _____

Spiritual Activity: _____

My Emotions Today: ❏ Happy ❏ Sad ❏ Stressed

Day/Date:

Breakfast: _____

Lunch: _____

Dinner: _____

Snacks: _____

GROUP	FRUITS	VEGETABLES	GRAINS	MEAT & BEANS	MILK	OILS
Goal Amount						
Estimate Your Total						
Total Calories						

Physical Activity: _____

Steps/Miles/Minutes: _____

Spiritual Activity: _____

My Emotions Today: ❏ Happy ❏ Sad ❏ Stressed

Day/Date:

Breakfast: _____

Lunch: _____

Dinner: _____

Snacks: _____

GROUP	FRUITS	VEGETABLES	GRAINS	MEAT & BEANS	MILK	OILS
Goal Amount						
Estimate Your Total						
Total Calories						

Physical Activity: _____

Steps/Miles/Minutes: _____

Spiritual Activity: _____

My Emotions Today: ❏ Happy ❏ Sad ❏ Stressed

Day/Date:

Live It Tracker

Name: _____ Date: _____ Week #: _____

Loss/gain _____ lbs. Calorie Range: _____ My food goal for the week: _____

_____

Activity Level: None, < 30 min/day, 30-60 min/day, 60+ min/day   My activity goal for the week: _____

My spiritual goal for the week: _____

Group	Daily Calories							
	1300-1400	1500-1600	1700-1800	1900-2000	2100-2200	2300-2400	2500-2600	2700-2800
Fruits	1.5-2 c.	1.5-2 c.	1.5-2 c.	2-2.5 c.	2-2.5 c.	2.5-3.5 c.	3.5-4.5 c.	3.5-4.5 c.
Vegetables	1.5-2 c.	2-2.5 c.	2.5-3 c.	2.5-3 c.	3-3.5 c.	3.5-4.5 c.	4.5-5 c.	4.5-5 c.
Grains	5 oz-eq.	5-6 oz-eq.	6-7 oz-eq.	6-7 oz-eq.	7-8 oz-eq.	8-9 oz-eq.	9-10 oz-eq.	10-11 oz-eq.
Meat & Beans	4 oz-eq.	5 oz-eq.	5-5.5 oz-eq.	5.5-6.5 oz-eq.	6.5-7 oz-eq.	7-7.5 oz-eq.	7-7.5 oz-eq.	7.5-8 oz-eq.
Milk	2-3 c.	3 c.	3 c.	3 c.	3 c.	3 c.	3 c.	3 c.
Healthy Oils	4 tsp.	5 tsp.	5 tsp.	6 tsp.	6 tsp.	7 tsp.	8 tsp.	8 tsp.

Day/Date:

Breakfast: _____
Lunch: _____
Dinner: _____
Snacks: _____

GROUP	FRUITS	VEGETABLES	GRAINS	MEAT & BEANS	MILK	OILS
Goal Amount						
Estimate Your Total						
Total Calories						

Physical Activity: _____ Spiritual Activity: _____
Steps/Miles/Minutes: _____ My Emotions Today: ❑ Happy   ❑ Sad   ❑ Stressed

Day/Date:

Breakfast: _____
Lunch: _____
Dinner: _____
Snacks: _____

GROUP	FRUITS	VEGETABLES	GRAINS	MEAT & BEANS	MILK	OILS
Goal Amount						
Estimate Your Total						
Total Calories						

Physical Activity: _____ Spiritual Activity: _____
Steps/Miles/Minutes: _____ My Emotions Today: ❑ Happy   ❑ Sad   ❑ Stressed

Day/Date:

Breakfast: _____
Lunch: _____
Dinner: _____
Snacks: _____

GROUP	FRUITS	VEGETABLES	GRAINS	MEAT & BEANS	MILK	OILS
Goal Amount						
Estimate Your Total						
Total Calories						

Physical Activity: _____ Spiritual Activity: _____
Steps/Miles/Minutes: _____ My Emotions Today: ❑ Happy   ❑ Sad   ❑ Stressed

Day/Date:

Breakfast: _____
Lunch: _____
Dinner: _____
Snacks: _____

GROUP	FRUITS	VEGETABLES	GRAINS	MEAT & BEANS	MILK	OILS
Goal Amount						
Estimate Your Total						
Total Calories						

Physical Activity: _____   Spiritual Activity: _____
Steps/Miles/Minutes: _____   My Emotions Today: ❑ Happy ❑ Sad ❑ Stressed

---

Day/Date:

Breakfast: _____
Lunch: _____
Dinner: _____
Snacks: _____

GROUP	FRUITS	VEGETABLES	GRAINS	MEAT & BEANS	MILK	OILS
Goal Amount						
Estimate Your Total						
Total Calories						

Physical Activity: _____   Spiritual Activity: _____
Steps/Miles/Minutes: _____   My Emotions Today: ❑ Happy ❑ Sad ❑ Stressed

---

Day/Date:

Breakfast: _____
Lunch: _____
Dinner: _____
Snacks: _____

GROUP	FRUITS	VEGETABLES	GRAINS	MEAT & BEANS	MILK	OILS
Goal Amount						
Estimate Your Total						
Total Calories						

Physical Activity: _____   Spiritual Activity: _____
Steps/Miles/Minutes: _____   My Emotions Today: ❑ Happy ❑ Sad ❑ Stressed

---

Day/Date:

Breakfast: _____
Lunch: _____
Dinner: _____
Snacks: _____

GROUP	FRUITS	VEGETABLES	GRAINS	MEAT & BEANS	MILK	OILS
Goal Amount						
Estimate Your Total						
Total Calories						

Physical Activity: _____   Spiritual Activity: _____
Steps/Miles/Minutes: _____   My Emotions Today: ❑ Happy ❑ Sad ❑ Stressed

let's count our miles!

Join the 100-Mile Club this Session

Can't walk that mile yet? Don't be discouraged! There are exercises you can do to strengthen your body and burn those extra calories. Keep a record on your Live It Tracker of the number of minutes you do these common physical activities, convert those minutes to miles following the chart below, and then mark off each mile you have completed on the chart found on the back of the back cover. Report your miles to your 100-Mile Club representative when you first arrive each week. Remember, you are not competing with anyone else . . . just yourself. Your job is to strive to reach 100 miles before the last meeting in this session. You can do it—just keep on moving!

Walking

slowly, 2 MPH	30 min.	= 156 cal.	= 1 mile
moderately, 3 MPH	20 min.	= 156 cal.	= 1 mile
very briskly, 4 MPH	15 min.	= 156 cal.	= 1 mile
speed walking	10 min.	= 156 cal.	= 1 mile
up stairs	13 min.	= 159 cal.	= 1 mile

Running/Jogging

	10 min.	= 156 cal.	= 1 mile

Cycling Outdoors

slowly, <10 MPH	20 min.	= 156 cal.	= 1 mile
light effort, 10-12 MPH	12 min.	= 156 cal.	= 1 mile
moderate effort, 12-14 MPH	10 min.	= 156 cal.	= 1 mile
vigorous effort, 14-16 MPH	7.5 min.	= 156 cal.	= 1 mile
very fast, 16-19 MPH	6.5 min.	= 152 cal.	= 1 mile

Sports Activities

Playing tennis (singles)	10 min.	= 156 cal.	= 1 mile
Swimming			
light to moderate effort	11 min.	= 152 cal.	= 1 mile
fast, vigorous effort	7.5 min.	= 156 cal.	= 1 mile
Softball	15 min.	= 156 cal.	= 1 mile
Golf	20 min.	= 156 cal	= 1 mile
Rollerblading	6.5 min.	= 152 cal.	= 1 mile
Ice skating	11 min.	= 152 cal.	= 1 mile

Jumping rope	7.5 min.	= 156 cal.	= 1 mile
Basketball	12 min.	= 156 cal.	= 1 mile
Soccer (casual)	15 min.	= 159 cal.	= 1 mile

Around the House

Mowing grass	22 min.	= 156 cal.	= 1 mile
Mopping, sweeping, vacuuming	19.5 min.	= 155 cal.	= 1 mile
Cooking	40 min.	= 160 cal.	= 1 mile
Gardening	19 min.	= 156 cal.	= 1 mile
Housework (general)	35 min.	= 156 cal.	= 1 mile
Ironing	45 min.	= 153 cal.	= 1 mile
Raking leaves	25 min.	= 150 cal.	= 1 mile
Washing car	23 min.	= 156 cal.	= 1 mile
Washing dishes	45 min.	= 153 cal.	= 1 mile

At the Gym

Stair machine	8.5 min.	= 155 cal.	= 1 mile
Stationary bike			
slowly, 10 MPH	30 min.	= 156 cal.	= 1 mile
moderately, 10-13 MPH	15 min.	= 156 cal.	= 1 mile
vigorously, 13-16 MPH	7.5 min.	= 156 cal.	= 1 mile
briskly, 16-19 MPH	6.5 min.	= 156 cal.	= 1 mile
Elliptical trainer	12 min.	= 156 cal.	= 1 mile
Weight machines (used vigorously)	13 min.	= 152 cal.	= 1 mile
Aerobics			
low impact	15 min.	= 156 cal.	= 1 mile
high impact	12 min.	= 156 cal.	= 1 mile
water	20 min.	= 156 cal.	= 1 mile
Pilates	15 min.	= 156 cal.	= 1 mile
Raquetball (casual)	15 min.	= 159 cal.	= 1 mile
Stretching exercises	25 min.	= 150 cal.	= 1 mile
Weight lifting (also works for weight machines used moderately or gently)	30 min.	= 156 cal.	= 1 mile

Family Leisure

Playing piano	37 min.	= 155 cal.	= 1 mile
Jumping rope	10 min.	= 152 cal.	= 1 mile
Skating (moderate)	20 min.	= 152 cal.	= 1 mile
Swimming			
moderate	17 min.	= 156 cal.	= 1 mile
vigorous	10 min.	= 148 cal.	= 1 mile
Table tennis	25 min.	= 150 cal.	= 1 mile
Walk/run/play with kids	25 min.	= 150 cal.	= 1 mile